How to Build a Better Human

How to Build a Better Human

An Ethical Blueprint

Gregory E. Pence

ROWMAN & LITTLEFIELD PUBLISHERS, INC.
Lanham • Boulder • New York • Toronto • Plymouth, UK

Published by Rowman & Littlefield Publishers, Inc.
A wholly owned subsidiary of The Rowman & Littlefield Publishing Group, Inc.
4501 Forbes Boulevard, Suite 200, Lanham, Maryland 20706
www.rowman.com

10 Thornbury Road, Plymouth PL6 7PP, United Kingdom

British Library Cataloguing in Publication Information Available

Library of Congress Cataloging-in-Publication Data

Pence, Gregory E.
How to build a better human : an ethical blueprint / Gregory E. Pence.
p. cm.
Includes bibliographical references and index.
ISBN 978-1-4422-1762-1 (cloth : alk. paper) -- ISBN 978-1-4422-1764-5 (electronic)
I. Title. [DNLM: 1. Biomedical Enhancement--ethics. 2. Bioethical Issues. 3. Genetic Counseling--ethics. W 82]
174.2--dc23

2012017542

The paper used in this publication meets the minimum requirements of American National Standard for Information Sciences Permanence of Paper for Printed Library Materials, ANSI/NISO Z39.48-1992.

Printed in the United States of America

Contents

PART III: CHANGING HUMAN NATURE?

Acknowledgments

This book had a long genesis. I presented parts of it as talks at Yale University at a meeting of the World Transhumanist Association, at talks to the Neurobiology Department at Northwestern University, at Agnes Scott College in Atlanta, GA, in Lausanne, Switzerland, in the Distinguished Anniversary lecture at the Federal University of Minas Gerais in Brazil, as the Henry Smits Lecture at Truman State University in Kirksville, MO, and as a keynote speaker in 2008 for the Mississippi Philosophical Association. I gave the first version of this talk to the University Honors Program at UAB.

I thank the best man at my wedding, Alfred Garwood, whom I first met in graduate school nearly forty years ago and who is still a good friend, for many conversations and for his careful, sympathetic comments on this book. His thoughtful entering into this manuscript with his whole mind and heart powerfully changed it for the better. My mother, Louise Pence, read several versions of this book and always supported it, even if she did persistently keep asking when it was ever going to appear.

Writing is a lonely business. Through this business, the physician-writer Abraham Verghese has been a comforting, supportive voice, and I am in his debt in many ways.

In the summer of 2008, I had four able research assistants, all members of the Early Medical School Acceptance Program at UAB: Anand Bosmia, Christina Ho, Jennifer Ghandhi, and Khushboo Jhala. They tracked down articles and references, helped proofread and edit the book, and helped sustain me in the writing of it. As usual, my students gave me more than I gave them. Mrs. Minnie Randle, who was named employee-of-the-month at UAB that same summer of 2008, deserves that honor and more, in part for all her help in writing this book and with other projects.

Later in 2008, medical student Freedom Jackson was my able research assistant in a Special Topics course. Freedom's prior decade of experience in a famous Birmingham law firm proved especially valuable to me.

In the summer of 2010, EMSAP students Allen Young, Michelle Chang, and Rachael Rosales helped on this book, serving as my summer interns, and subjecting my own writing to their rigorous proofing for sense, grammar, and typos. In spring 2012, my EMSAP students Amanda Allredge and Brynna Paulukaitis proofed the manuscript, discovering numerous small errors and really improving the flow of the material. Never has a professor had better assistants, and I am grateful for their persistent efforts.

In 2011, Dennis Watts—retired from the Department of Medicine at UAB—and some of his family kindly read a version of this manuscript and offered great comments. I am in their debt. My retired colleague, G. Lynn Stephens, read my chapter on professional athletes and steroids and corrected several errors of fact. Professors Tollefsbol and Bamman helped too.

UAB prides itself on being an interdisciplinary research university where interactions occur. Sometimes this is propaganda, sometimes mere hope, but in my case, it has been a dream. No philosopher or bioethicist has profited more than I from hearing talks in other fields and by scientists far afield from philosophy. Even basic lectures in our medical school on seemingly unrelated topics later bore fruit in this book. You never know when a fact will touch a concept.

Preface

For folic acid, the B vitamin now added to cereals and wheats in North America, the breakthrough came around 1991. Until that year, scientists suspected, but could not prove, that women who took folic acid during pregnancy dramatically reduced neural tube defects in newborns. When the neural tube doesn't close properly, the result in fetal development can be such defects as spina bifida, an opening in the spine that causes lower paralysis, or anencephaly, a complete lack of higher parts of the brain,

Britain had long suffered a relatively high rate of such defects as well. As a result, its Medical Research Council started a randomized clinical trial in 1983 to see if women who had borne such a child could take folic acid to lessen their chances of having another.[1] By 1991, researchers saw a 71 percent reduction of neural tube defects, and the Research Council began to encourage all pregnant women to take folic acid.

In 1998, Canada began adding folic acid to enriched pasta, white flour, and cereals; by 2002, it had halved its rate of neural tube defects.[2].Eventually the United States did the same, but how and why folic acid came to be required in American cereals is a long story that I'll tell later.

Today, folic acid stands as a great success story of North American medicine. It's also a story of how humans can ethically enhance themselves by creating better babies from conception.

The cases that this book describes show that humans, if they are careful and rational, can enhance themselves, and do so ethically. That is, we can utilize genetics, biotechnology, and medicine in safe, *ethical* ways. For humans, enhancement is not the enemy of the ethical.

I define "human enhancement" broadly as any attempt to improve humans, whether in a particular life or for future humans, whether in utero or late in life through drugs, whether incrementally by adding vitamins to cereal or suddenly by giving everyone smart phones.

It may surprise fundamentalists that medicine has been quietly enhancing people for decades and has neither become Nazi-like, nor has it, for the most part, seriously harmed anyone. It's time that we ignore Alarmists and think about human enhancement in public, practical, serious ways.

What are those ways? Well, one of those ways concerns how we "do" ethics. We shouldn't lump all cases of enhancement together any more than we should lump all kinds of technology together. As Aristotle said, we need to treat different kinds of cases separately. If we don't, bad things happen.

We also need to transcend the two common frame stories of bioethics: bioconservative alarmism and uncritical enthusiasm. Neither does justice to the complexities of medicine nor to the real problems of enhancing humans.

But we need to get going. By 2012, we've had a half-century of bioethics (dating its start from the 1962 God Committee). It's time that bioethics became part of the solution, not the problem, in making better humans.

NOTES

1. Susan White Junod, "Folic Acid Fortification: Fact and Folly," Update, the bimonthly publication of the Food and Drug Law Institute. http://www.fda.gov/oc/history/makinghistory/folicacid.html
2. De Wals, "Reduction in Neural Tube Defects after Folic Acid Fortification in Canada," New England Journal of Medicine 357, July 12, 2007, 135-142.

PART I

COMPETENT ADULTS
ENHANCING THEMSELVES

Chapter One

What if Your Virtual Life Surpasses Your Real Life?

In a year in the future sooner than we think, Josh walks to a skyscraper, takes an elevator to the thirtieth floor, enters a familiar room, lies down in a special bed, pays a fee, enters a password, and attaches a thick cable to a bioport—one surgically implanted behind his ear. His wetware connects to Virtual Life, an artificial world far better than any we know today and where Josh enjoys simulated experiences. For the next few hours, Josh's body will be monitored by attendants who are supervised by an on-site physician.

Josh soon starts to hike up the Himalayas in Nepal. His hike there feels so life-like, so interactive, and so tactile that for Josh, his experience feels as good as actual hiking. Sometimes it is even better, because these hikes lack freezing rain or slippery rocks.

On this day, Josh starts at the Buddhist monastery at Kathmandu and inhales cool, clean air, then feels a little altitude sickness. He crosses a stream of ice-fed water and feels the cold. Turning back, he sees a stunning view of the valley, revealing a great river below. Josh travels here for four hours. His trip concluded, Josh remembers his exhilarating adventure and can't wait for the next. Despite a substantial deposit, he instantly books another.

In a cubicle near him, Erica lies in a similar bed, but she chooses simulated sex. For multiple reasons, including a demanding job, an off-putting personality, and a body that does not conform to cultural ideals of femininity, Erica's real-life experiences have failed to satisfy her. In Virtual Life, she finds what she wants.

We need not trouble ourselves about what kind of fantasy Erica has. We know that people have fantasies about sex and that such fantasies differ because of gender, sexual orientation, upbringing, random associations, and culture.

It is important that Erica's experience is a simulacrum, not reality. Everyone in Virtual Life does what Erica wants. That, of course, is false in reality. Virtual Life is not a massively multiplayer online role-playing game (MMORPG) where Erica would interact with virtual personas of real people. In Virtual Life, Erica only interacts with virtual people.

For our discussion, the premises about Virtual Life that matter are that (1) fantasies can be satisfied, and (2) because no other real people are involved, no one (other than Josh or Erica) can be directly harmed. It is also important for Josh and Erica that, no matter which fantasy each explores, he or she is completely safe.

Is Virtual Life farfetched? Not at all. In a recent issue of *New York Magazine* devoted to pornography and the Internet, many people admitted to frequenting high-quality Internet pornographic sites, some several times a day. Some also visited interactive sites where actors were paid to act sexually. Some people liked on-line sex more than sex with real people.

The article in *New York* described the billions of dollars in revenue that the Internet-based pornography industry generates, how demand for such services historically drives innovation for better forms of broadcast, and how owners anticipate future enhancements.

In the ethics of human enhancement, the topic of enhanced virtual experiences is a toddler among adults. Scholars in the literature typically discuss the effects of Cyborgian links to the Internet or brain-boosting drugs (both discussed later), but here we discuss enhanced virtual *experience*—the Internet version of the opium den.

The ethical issues raised by such experiences will be upon us sooner than we expect. In 1979, futurist and science fiction writer Arthur C. Clarke used a special satellite-linked phone from Sri Lanka to talk to a reporter in America. Similarly in 1980, physician-writer Michael Crichton had explorers in *Congo* phone home from the jungles of Africa to America via a satellite-linked phone. At the time, such devices so exceeded expectations that these writers could mention them to impress their readers. Now they are dated. Today, *anybody* can use a cell phone to call anywhere on the planet. Similarly, high-definition television, once the purchase of the rich, has become the norm in developed countries. Technology moves fast, especially technology that people desire. How might it do so with Virtual Life? Consider the creation of dialysis machines around 1960.

At its inception, physicians had to connect new catheters to the patient's veins and arteries each time he or she underwent dialysis. Because of bruising and infection, the catheters wouldn't stay in place, and after a few weeks, the patient looked like Frankenstein's monster, with stitches and bruises over his body.

Around 1962, Seattle physician Belding Scribner created a permanent, indwelling Teflon shunt, similar to a spigot, so nurses could connect and reconnect the same catheters for withdrawing and returning blood, making viable long-term kidney dialysis. (In so doing, Scribner created a classic problem in bioethics: Who shall live when not all can?) The Teflon surface prevented surface antigens from causing the patient's immune system to reject the shunt. Over the years, surgeons created better, longer-lasting shunts and today, patients may live on dialysis for decades.

The effectiveness of synthetic connections to veins today may be as high as 50 percent, compared to 85 percent for using veins from a patient's own body. The major problem is formation of clots on synthetic connections.

Surgeons overcame these problems with a technique called *endothelial seeding*. The endothelium refers to the layer of flat cells lining the closed spaces of the body, such as the inside of blood vessels, lymphatic vessels, and the heart. In contrast, the epithelium, the outside layer of cells, covers all the free, open surfaces of the body, including the skin and mucous membranes.

Endothelial seeding exemplifies the field of tissue engineering, in which inorganic and biological materials fuse to replace, repair, and aid parts of the human body. Tissue engineering differs from regenerative medicine, where the body's own adult or embryonic stem cells are grown to generate new cells as replacements for dysfunctional cells.

Endothelial cells of the patient grown in culture can be seeded onto a variety of surfaces to produce an intervening layer. Special techniques in biotechnology can seed endothelial cells onto filters, grafts, tubes, as well as other artificial biomaterials and prostheses. [1] Scientists get good results by growing such cells under glass from fatty tissue and transferring them to grow on some artificial material. In Phase III clinical trials, where benefit to patients is expected, surgeons use vascular endothelial growth factor 2 (VEGF-2) to facilitate the connections. [2]

In the near future, a new Belding Scribner will create an indwelling bioport, perhaps with endothelial seeding, through which the brain can connect wirelessly to an external personal computer and the Internet. That connection will be a quantum leap in the brain's history. At once, almost every human will radically increase his available knowledge, memory, and ability to calculate. It will enable each human to cooperate, communicate, and socialize with any other group of humans on a military team, in a family, on an inspection team, or in a university class. It will open the door to Virtual Life.

Farfetched? Consider that scientists recently implanted a freckle-sized grid containing one hundred tiny electrodes over a patch of cells in a monkey's brain. Researchers tied down the monkey's arms and wired the electrodes to a mechanical arm that could bring food to the monkey's mouth.

Previous experiments demonstrated that human spinal cord patients could move a cursor on a computer screen with brain waves and that monkeys could use brain waves to move a robotic hand. Solely with their thoughts, the monkeys quickly learned to adjust the prosthesis for size and stickiness of bits of food. Amazingly, after being taught with biofeedback, each monkey mastered his new arm in just a few days. The *New York Times* called this "the most striking demonstration to date of brain-machine interface technology." [3]

The problems of this interface resemble those before Scribner perfected his shunt: after a few months, the electrodes degrade and the equipment needed to transmit the wireless signal needs improvement, *but these are solvable problems.* It takes no great genius to see that future researchers will improve the wireless connections that allow monkeys to act with external prostheses.

If this happens, the ethical transition from therapy to enhancement will be quick. Who would deny quadriplegic patients implanted electrodes that signal wirelessly to a laptop? So many patients retain active minds even after lungs, kidneys, or hearts give out and limit physical activities. Even if medicine cannot restore their ability to walk, new wetware connections could give them another twenty years of mental life. Can you say *Avatar*?

It's plausible to imagine wetware connections to parts of the brain that control appendages, genitals, elimination, and eating. It's plausible that we will soon enter a virtual, 3-D world in high-definition color that allows any fantasy to come true: not only simulated travel or sex, but also simulated acting in *MacBeth* or quarterbacking for the Dallas Cowboys.

The question of such a Virtual Life recalls one raised by philosopher Robert Nozick and his famous Experience Machine.[4] Nozick premised that you had to make a devil's bargain—once you entered the fantasy, you believed it was your real life and you forgot your original bargain. You opted for an upbeat version of the Matrix, but before you downloaded into it, you had to drink the waters of forgetfulness.

Nozick's premise should be rejected for two reasons: first, the technology to fool yourself totally and forever seems too far-off to be practical; second, why opt out forever? What if your body got appendicitis or a high fever? You want to be around to decide what to do for it, lest it die.

Let us assume more practically that we can enter Virtual Life, but we can exit it at any time. In other words, at some level we are conscious that we're in Virtual Life.

So let's assume that it's a great world, far superior to anything yet conceived, and for most people, far better than their real lives. Suppose that in real life you work on an assembly line cutting up chickens in a cold factory. But in Virtual Life, you are a sorcerer-baker and your superb pies attract satisfied centaurs, dwarves, and kings. This makes you quite happy and you have great interactions, especially with the male dwarves.

Which brings us to some philosophical questions about Virtual Life: does it exhibit bad values to live in it? Is it immoral to live in it? Moreover, should public policy encourage life there, e.g., for the unemployed or disabled?

A basic criticism is that what's bad about Virtual Life is *that it's not real*, that all your conquests, victories, self-esteem, prizes are fake. Your experiences exist only in your head and in the program of the computer.

In reply, to argue, "Real experiences are better than simulated experiences because they're real," is to beg the question of what makes reality so great, anyway.

Accept the premise that Virtual Life delivers experiences of travel, sex, eating, and competition as good as their real-life counterparts. Given that premise, consider a crucial philosophical question: are you *cheating yourself* of something valuable by spending your free time in Virtual Life?

Answering this question is not easy and any good answer will have different parts and will vary according to the example. Consider sex. If someone claims that virtual sex is as good as actual sex, this forces us to think about what makes sexual relations good.

One traditional answer is that sexual relations lead to children. St. Augustine said God permitted married couples to have sex to create children, but only for this reason. Once they had the children they wanted, the permission was revoked.

Virtually no one believes this anymore, even the Catholic Church, which now teaches that loving marriages should include sexual relations even after child-bearing has passed. Moreover, scientists have separated sexual relations from reproduction from two directions: because of contraception and abortion, people can have sex without reproducing, and because of advances in assisted reproduction, people can reproduce without having sex.

If we sever the link between sex and reproduction, then the probability of good virtual sex forces us to ask the question of what makes sex with a real person good. One traditional answer is that sex with a real person involves intimacy. Intimacy includes many things: communication, friendship, and relationships.

But some people notoriously desire sex without relationships or intimacy. Are they perverts?

In his autobiographical *My Own Country,* Abraham Verghese, an AIDS doctor in rural Tennessee, visits a gay bar and observes the scene. He later muses that gay men act as straight men would act if they could find women willing to have anonymous, quick sex most nights. Is this what Virtual Life will give men? And for the first time in female history, will it equalize women the same way?

There is an elephant in this virtual room, and he's the traditionalist who bellows, "What's wrong with simulated travel or simulated sex is that IT'S NOT REAL!! IT'S FAKE." The continuing objection here is that if your emotional center becomes living in Virtual Life, then you've lost your real life. You've cheated yourself of real experiences in a life. You're not authentic and your experiences are no more substantial than the pleasant dreams of an opium addict.

There is some truth in this claim. If we think about ideal sexual relations, whether in a monogamous relationship or otherwise, sexual experiences with real people bring other goods that make the intrinsic desirability of (what Alvin Goldman famously called) "plain sex" better.[5] These goods include ongoing relations, knowledge of a partner, and trust.

On the other hand, some people prefer sexual variety, and Virtual Life can deliver that. More importantly, some people may decide that they are unlikely to have ideal sex, or even good sex, or perhaps, any real consensual sex at all, and therefore Virtual Sex is right for them.

Consider the paraplegic in a wheelchair, the elderly widower who is still functional, and someone whose occupation forces him to live alone (a fire ranger in an isolated tower in Montana). For such people, it is difficult to see why Virtual Sex is bad.

Suppose Erica, in real life, is attracted to men who are abusive, alcoholics, or otherwise bad for her. In Virtual Life, she can have the sort of sex she wants without the dysfunctionality and still have male friends in the real world. Is that so terrible?

Consider Elaine, a worker laboring for minimum wage, barely making enough to pay her bills. On the rare times when Elaine has a few extra dollars, she can get drunk or instead spend an hour in Virtual Life—as she likes to do—floating down the Nile River as Queen Cleopatra. Assuming Elaine is monitored for medical problems, it is hard to see why virtual floating isn't a wiser choice than getting drunk. Indeed, if Elaine is pregnant, then Elaine is *obligated* to choose Virtual Life over drinking.

Objection: experiences in Virtual Life affect how one experiences the real world. If all one's relationships are great in Virtual Life, how will one fare in reality with real relationships, which notoriously go up and down? Will Virtual Life spoil the young for real life? Also, it's not completely true, as previously assumed, that "no one other than Josh or Erica" can be directly harmed in Virtual Life. What if their spouses or families suffer because Josh and Erica spend too much time there? Maybe it's not a direct harm, but it could still be substantial.

Notice that in the field of enhancement ethics, virtual experiences enhance mental life in a quite different sense than brain-boosting drugs enhance scores on college tests or enhance performance at work, for virtual experiences enhance *satisfaction*. Satisfaction is an intensely private, personal good.

Isn't that something a good society should foster? Is there anything wrong with doing so? After all, millions of humans have escaped into stories, movies, plays, television, novels, comics, or watching sports for centuries. Isn't it a good to have better escapes and more satisfaction?

The ethical theory of utilitarianism has a special problem explaining why life in Virtual Life is bad. Jeremy Bentham, the originator of utilitarianism, famously held with regard to pleasure, "Pushpin is as good as poetry," meaning that the lowbrow pleasures of bowling are just as good as the highbrow pleasures of poetry. For utilitarians such as Bentham, pleasure is pleasure and it's good to create more pleasure in the world. But if the pleasure of winning virtual combat is just as good as winning real combat, then utilitarians seem unable to object.

How might Virtual Life grab hold of people? Answer: through the door of therapy. Therapy is the door through which all enhancements traditionally enter. Breast construction came first for women after a mastectomy, later for healthy women who wanted larger or smaller breasts. Viagra was first used for men with sexual dysfunction, later for healthy men for enhanced function.

The first person to use a new exoskeleton was Yangchih Tan, a paraplegic since an accident in 1990 and who, using his new exoskeleton in late 2011, took 150 steps, his first in two decades.[6] Ekso Bionics of Berkeley, California hopes to perfect this exoskeleton soon.

Consider a paralyzed veteran who can't move his appendages, or a victim of locked-in-syndrome, a neurological condition resembling a persistent vegetative state, but in which a patient is actually aware and can blink. Virtual Life could be stupendous for them and enhance their lives. Is there anyone who could counter the gale storm of indignation of the paralyzed veteran's sister who wants Virtual Life for her brother? Who believes the country owes it to him for his sacrifice?

Other people will feel the same way. Woe be unto the Alarmist who blocks Sarah from helping her grandfather, who can hardly walk after his heart attack, from having Virtual Life, where he can be an eighteen-year-old young buck and sports hero. Who could be so cruel?

In short, needs of patients will trump sermons. Virtual Life will help the victims of the psychiatric locked-in-syndrome, the blind and deaf, the totally paralyzed, and others with active minds but dead bodies. Once it is perfected, it will enhance experience for all of us.

The military will utilize Virtual Life in training warriors for battle. What better place to see who is courageous, who is a leader, who is a sharpshooter, than in a life-like, three-dimensional battle?

Another elephant in the room in our discussion is addiction. What if the real danger is not the soma of *Brave New World*, but the psyche of Virtual Life? The question is not what if Virtual Life unleashes a previously unknown form of addiction but *when* will it do so and *how many* will be addicted. Most writing about addiction focuses on drugs, but what about addiction to life-expanding *experiences*?

If we grant the premise that Virtual Life could be as addictive as cocaine, bioconservatives correctly endorse regulation. Some people will be so vulnerable, so mentally or emotionally weak, that their vicarious lives will quickly overpower their own. Just as opium dens were banned for the public good, so may fantasy dens need to be banned for some.

Suppose your experiences in Virtual Life as a Knight at King Arthur's Round Table are so good that you neglect to pick up your child from school. If Virtual Life became so addictive as to cause such behaviors, especially in large numbers, then it would need to be regulated. People with obligations to children would need to prove they could handle Virtual Life or be limited to a few hours a day after their children were asleep.

Indeed, if we take the premise a little further and imagine that Virtual Life offers a life *twice as* satisfying as normal life, then we know people will not want to leave it. Then we know that we have Internet Soma.

One way that Virtual Life can be regulated, and which fiscal conservatives should endorse, is by cost. It will be expensive to hire the actors and actresses to do the voices and act out the scenarios that make Virtual Life feel real (this will also create employment for struggling actors). If an hour in Virtual Life costs the same as playing eighteen holes of golf, then most people could not afford to live there too much and would need to keep working to pay.

Nevertheless, I resist the idea that such a satisfying Virtual Life is *intrinsically bad*. Pleasure is good and a technology that allows more people to have more pleasure is good. Such technology should not be relegated in advance to the dustbin of moral condemnation.

What bothers me about continuous life in Virtual Life is that it seems dangerously close to pharmacological addiction and not having real friends, but only having friends on social networks over the Internet. (However, as one of my students objected, "Having only Facebook friends is better than having no friends at all.")

But when Virtual Life gets really good, some will decide that it's rational to live there as much as possible. Can this be defended?

I am not sure, but I believe it will come down to personal values. To say it's a matter of personal values is to say it shouldn't be made illegal to escape there. On the other hand, public policy doesn't need to subsidize it with a tax deduction and can tax it like alcohol or cigarettes.

Personally, I am a concrete, practically oriented person. Those who are escapists by nature might find Virtual Life compelling. For me, because Virtual Life is a fake world, it will always be less valuable than the real world. But I recognize that rational people will differ: their prospects might be worse than mine or their life in their part of the world might be so abysmal that Virtual Life looks great.

As with the other topics of this book, the time to think about these new issues is now, for they will come sooner than we think.

NOTES

1. U. S. Ryan and B. M. Olazabal, "Endothelial Seeding of Filters, Grafts, and Tubes."
http://www.springerlink.com/content/k1hh383322022651
2. http://www.bryantresearch.com/pdf/Phizer_june.pdf
   2. Holly Finn, "Meet the Real Bionic Man," *Wall Street Journal*, October 23, 2011, C1.
   3. Benedict Carey, "Monkeys Control Robotic Arm with their Thoughts," May 29, 2008, *New York Times*, A1.
   4. Robert Nozick, *Anarchy, State and Utopia* (New York: Basic Books, 1977), 45.
   5. Alan Goldman, "Plain Sex," *Philosophy and Public Affairs*, 6, no. 3 (Spring 1977), 267—87.
   6. Holly Finn, "Meet the Real Bionic Man," *Wall Street Journal*, October 23, 2011, C1.

Chapter Two

Lessons from the History of Bioethics

"Treat similar cases similarly; dissimilar cases dissimilarly."
—Aristotle, *Nichomachean Ethics*

Current discussion of enhancement of humans suffers from a depressing mistake that has infected bioethics for a half-century: lumping too many different kinds of cases together. Cases of human enhancement differ dramatically, just as do kinds of technology. Gene therapy on future generations of children does not raise the same issues as those of giving Ritalin to existing children. We should not lump the ethical issues of smart phones under technology as if they resembled those of nuclear energy.

In the history of bioethics, this lesson has been hard to learn. Consider death and dying. In 1975, twenty-one-year-old Karen Quinlan mixed alcohol with barbiturates and tranquilizers, causing her to fall into a persistent vegetative state. After months of hoping that she would emerge from her coma, her parents decided to remove her respirator so that she could pass away. A lower-court judge disagreed and the Quinlans appealed to the New Jersey Supreme Court.

The court's decision in 1976 granted her parents the right to remove the respirator, allegedly based on Karen's personal liberty to live as she chose. Tragically, for the next decades of law and bioethics, courts referred to Karen *as if she were a competent patient*, which she was not.

This decision mistakenly lumped together the liberty-rights of competent patients with those of families of incompetent patients, and all those with another kind of right, the rights of now-incompetent-but-formerly-competent patients. As we now know, these cases profoundly differ from one another.

The right to privacy most obviously applies to us as competent patients and to our rights to determine our own medical destinies. Ideally, our courts would have first laid out that right and then tackled other issues, such as those affecting incompetent patients. But life didn't give the court that choice, so the *Quinlan* court tackled incompetent patients first.

It took fifteen more years before the U. S. Supreme Court straightened things out in its 1990 *Cruzan* decision. Over those years, a dozen different state supreme courts issued a dozen different, often conflicting, decisions about rights of patients at the end of life. These courts sometimes erred in lumping competent patients with incompetent patients.

Like Karen Quinlan, Nancy Cruzan had been in a persistent vegetative state for many years. Unlike Karen, Nancy's case involved removing a feeding tube, not a respirator. *Cruzan* laid down an important theme in American law about rights of dying patients, and *did so by distinguishing two different kinds of cases.* As simple as that sounds, that Court took a gigantic step. Merely keeping different kinds of cases separate would go a long way in bioethics, law, and public policy toward exposing self-promoting Alarmists and toward seeing the real issues clearly.

Unlike the *Quinlan* decision, *Cruzan* involved the standards of evidence that should be met by families wishing to remove feeding tubes or respirators from incompetent relatives. With regard to incompetent patients, *Cruzan* held that a state could, but need not, pass a statute requiring the clear and convincing standard of evidence about what a *formerly competent* patient would have wanted done. [1]

Critics of Joseph and Julia Quinlan made a mistake when they compared the Quinlans' decision to remove Karen's respirator with the Nazis' secret killing of six million Jews. They grouped nonsensational cases with horrible ones, smearing all with the same paint.

Of great importance, *Cruzan* recognized a right of competent patients to refuse medical treatment, even if such refusal led directly to their deaths. For the first time, the *Cruzan* decision by the U.S. Supreme Court stated that the Constitution gave competent citizens unrestricted freedom to refuse medical support, even against wishes of physicians and even if such patients had previously said something different. In the end, decisions of competent patients trumped everything; states could erect no evidentiary barriers to the supremacy of such decisions.

Why was it so important to consider different kinds of cases separately? Consider the justification each case needs. It is much easier to know the wishes of competent patients and to know if they are ambivalent, steadfast, or wish to change their minds than it is to know the wishes of incompetent patients, where physicians cannot judge ambivalence, strength of conviction, or intelligence. Different family members may disagree about actions that are in the best interests of the incompetent patient, or what she would have wanted done. For these reasons, treating these kinds of cases differently, each with different standards of evidence, makes perfect sense.

Remember the lesson that the courts should have started with *competent* patients and first decided their rights at the end of life. In thinking about how to improve humans, we need not repeat the mistake of the past, so we will start with competent adults enhancing themselves.

Let's apply that lesson. Consider *Beyond Therapy*, the analysis of enhancement options by Leon Kass and the President's Council on Bioethics.[2] It does not open by discussing whether restrictions should be put on competent patients' decisions to enhance themselves. Instead, it jumps right into decisions by parents that affect babies and future children, and then lumps these with pre-implantation genetic diagnosis in embryos, giving short kids growth hormones, and selecting packages of specific traits for designer children. Not only do these three cases differ as much as enhancing oranges, elephants, and spaceships, they ignore the historical role of competent adults in voluntary, medical experimentation.

Now consider a second famous issue in bioethics, assisted reproduction, and how the same mistake occurred there. In the early 1970s, a British documentary about in vitro fertilization set its tone by opening with footage of an exploding atomic bomb. Following this sensationalistic image, Warren Kornberg, editor of *Science News*, actually wrote in 1969 that ethical questions about assisted reproduction, cloning, and human genetics weighed equally in importance with those raised by the proliferation of atomic bombs.[3]

And there you have the basic mistake. Kornberg lumped helping a husband and wife, who wanted to create a wanted child with their own sperm and egg with *Blade Runner* and *GATTACA*. As an ethical issue, helping couples create wanted children should be relatively minor, but preventing nuclear war ranks as one of our most profound ethical issues, comparable to reducing the spread of HIV. It grabbed attention to compare IVF to nuclear war, but it did so in a confused, feverish way.

From the late 1950s to the mid-1970s, Yale Professor of Religious Studies Paul Ramsey and University of Chicago biochemist and physician Leon Kass most influenced the public in just these ways and, in doing so, became quite famous.[4] Ramsey and Kass ran together artificial insemination, in vitro fertilization, egg donation, surrogate mothers, cloning, and genetic engineering, condemning them all. Neither had any sympathy for the view that IVF, donation of sperm, egg transfer, or surrogacy might give infertile couples the child they desired.

Thirty years after Louise Brown's birth through IVF in 1978, millions of people worldwide have used assisted reproduction and now happily raise children. Assisted reproduction continues to be one of the fastest-growing, happiest sectors of medicine, being truly *pro-life* in ways that make theocons shudder. Alarmists still claim that IVF will make the sky fall, but millions of infertile couples ignore them.

Critics also categorized in vitro fertilization with cloning humans, and confused *coerced* conception with *chosen* conception. This fuzzy thinking blinded them to the desire of infertile couples for a child. When the government banned federal funding of research on human embryos, clinics financed such research with patients' fees, bypassing IRB's. Freed from bureaucratic obstacles and fueled by such fees, assisted reproduction took off.

In retrospect, the hysteria about assisted reproduction added up to *nonsense*. In almost all cases, the new techniques merely helped infertile couples along a bit. It's not as if scientists had created artificial sperm from chemicals.

Alarmists ran all these cases together, as well as two other different things: parental choice with state coercion, and a couple's preferences with Eugenics. When Alarmists resort to the same tricks, can we learn from history and resist their dire prophecies? Rather than running cases together and over-generalizing, we usually need to *downsize* the bioethical problem. When a new form of assisted reproduction comes along, we should reject statements such as "the fate of human nature is at stake," and substitute, "this is another small step in helping couples have the kids they want." In reality, it's the downsized problem that confronts physicians, not the choice to alter human nature.

Let us now turn our history of bioethics to our third topic, genetic engineering. Alarmists hurled the "playing God" charge not only about creating babies, but also about creating new combinations of genes. We can infer from the clichéd titles of not one but two books published in 1977. *Playing God* by journalist June Goodfield raised alarms about scientists tinkering with genes, DNA, and as her subtitle says, the "genetic engineering and the manipulation of life."[5] In that same year, bestselling Alarmist Jeremy Rifkin, together with Pastor Ted Howard, published *Who Should Play God? : The artificial creation of life and what it means for the future of the human race.*[6]

For forty years, Alarmists hurled the thought-stopping phrase "genetic engineering" against geneticists. Always Alarmist, this cliché rarely enlightens. It always predicts genetic doom and usually accompanies other phrases such as, "Medicine is changing faster than our wisdom," or "Science is changing faster than our ability to understand these changes."

Some past predictions amuse us now. In the summer of 1965, a molecular biologist on the staff of Rockefeller University, Rollin Hotchkiss, predicted to three thousand biologists at a meeting of the American Institute of Biological Sciences that "in five years" parents would be able to order children with blonde hair, blue eyes, and fair skin.[7] He described the process of "genetic engineering" as changing the hereditary traits of cells by introducing new genes. Hotchkiss went on to describe how a dictator might want to use genetic engineering and how the future implications were like "the revolution set in motion by the atomic bomb." Here again lies a gigantic category mistake. He noted that the first step would involve genetic intervention to fight disease, probably by using viruses.

Six months later on New Year's Day 1966, Nobel Prize-winning biologist F. M. Burnett urged a moratorium on genetic research on humans.[8] James Shannon, the director of the National Institutes of Health from 1955 to 1968, countered that genetic engineering could prevent inherited diseases, but Alarmists had set the tone.[9]

Critics of genetic engineering always hopped from one kind of case to another: from allowing parents and physicians to choose against, say, a child with a neural tube defect to allowing parents to choose to only have perfect children, from allowing choice to being coerced into accepting the Aryan ideal. In this mistake, Alarmists assumed that parents would be unable to distinguish the two kinds of cases or would not strenuously resist such control.

In any discussion of human enhancement, we should first divide our cases into the appropriate classes with their appropriate standards of evidence. Not doing so is exactly the mistake of Alarmists, who get themselves worked up over people who want to experiment on themselves and who act as if such self-experimentation is morally the same as experimenting on vulnerable babies. It is not.

A second lesson from the history of bioethics concerns the two frame stories by which bioethicists discuss new technology. A frame for a picture sets the limits of what can be shown and determines how the picture is revealed, and thus seen, by the audience. Frames become familiar to viewers, or readers, because they allow us to predict the outcome. Mark Twain famously used the frame story of the backwoods rube who is smarter than he seems and who exploits the smugness of stupid urbanites.

In bioethics, one frame story is *Alarmism* and it is fueled by bioconservatism. This story warns that it is hubris for humans to try to enhance their biological natures. When hubris tempts humans to act as gods, the gods strike them down, inflicting war, infectious diseases, revolution, or death.

The second frame for biotechnology is *Enthusiasm*, which I use in the old sense of David Hume's *History of England*. This frame story is most often used by transhumanism. This story claims that humans should attempt to enhance their nature. This position could well have sprung up during the Enlightenment, when educated people had passionate faith in science. The co-discoverer of the structure of DNA, James Watson, supports this position, as have people famous in the history of eugenics, such as Francis Galton and J. B. S. Haldane.[10] More recently, UCLA bioethicist Gregory Stock defends this position, as does English bioethicist John Harris in two books,[11] as well as James Hughes, Ramez Naam, and Nick Bostrom.[12]

The Alarmist frame story has been the most publicized, especially by public intellectuals. Since his 1970 essay "Making Babies" in *Atlantic*, Leon Kass has attacked unnatural biotechnology. He has opposed in vitro fertilization, surrogate gestation, embryonic cloning, reproductive cloning, and using Prozac.

As chair of George W. Bush's Council on Bioethics, Kass in 2003 wrote *Beyond Therapy: Biotechnology and the Pursuit of Happiness*, which opposed all attempts at human enhancement. Although it's the official report of the entire council, every page bears the stamp of Kass' writing. *Beyond Therapy* says that making our bodies stronger and longer-lived will turn our bodies into mere tools. As such, we will come to "despise" our given bodies. If we continue down this path, we will lose "who we are"—our human identity—and become something worse.

Bill McKibben, an Alarmist and naturalist, writes in *Enough!* that biotechnology has gone too far with assisted reproduction, genetically modified food, and cloning. We should strive, as Joni Mitchell famously sang, "to get back to the garden." McKibben, a modern Rousseau who got his start writing for the urbane *New Yorker*, implies that civilization is artificial, corruptive, and unhealthy, including the science that generates the modern world. As a champion of organic farming, Slow Food, and sustainable living, McKibben opposes enhancing humans. (Presumably, he will never get the *New Yorker* wirelessly or read it on a Kindle.)

Simplistic worldviews will not capture the best ethical analysis of various kinds of enhancement. Why? Because for a particular kind of enhancement, many different values (or what law professors call "interests") will compete, and we can predict that no simplistic position will be fair to all interests.

Digging into these frames reveals presumptions about why it is good or bad to enhance humans. For most bioconservatives, their primordial opposition stems from a religious worldview (whether they admit it or not) where humans are seen as imperfect creatures created by a perfect, omniscient deity. If you accept the premise that human nature is fallen, then it follows that humans will go wrong in trying to improve their natures. If you accept the premise that humans are made as they are for a reason, then not only does it make no sense to change them, it would be *wrong* to change them. In so doing, you would disrespect the gift of the Giver. If you believe that something Higher made each child as he is for a special reason, it's blasphemous to think that his parents could have chosen him to be healthier, smarter, or happier.

On the other hand, if you take the transhumanist position, and if you believe that humans are good, then the default position should be that humans must continuously try to enhance themselves. Medicine should not be a reluctant partner to enhancement, but a cheerleader. German medicine under the Nazi regime makes us cautious about this last statement.

Transhumanists tend to be uncritical champions of new technologies in medicine. A good example is their early embrace of robotic surgery, e.g., for prostatectomies or removal of gall bladders. Only long-term evidence will prove that robot-assisted surgery beats a sure human hand, and some anecdotal evidence already suggests that it does not. Simply adopting an attitude of acceptance to new things is not always wise.

In the last decades, transhumanists have been too enthusiastic about gene therapy. As I'll explain later, gene therapy has been a disaster, and we're nowhere near ready to do it routinely. "Genetic engineering," or gene enhancement of humans, is so far away from being safe that self-confident predictions about it in the past now seem laughable. We must be careful not to repeat the mistakes of gene therapy with stem cells and some forms of organic self-medication.

Unless overwhelming evidence can be marshalled for a particular attempt at enhancement, the default position for bioconservatives is a ban. In the debate about genetically modified food, bioconservative Europeans adopted the Precautionary Principle, meaning that they won't allow genetically modified food to be sold inside Europe until there is evidence beyond a reasonable doubt—an extraordinarily high standard—that such foods are safe. A similar view can be argued about abortion, that because you might be mistaken and because a human life might be at stake, you should always err on the side of life.

For transhumanists, the default position is to allow anything. In this regard, it is like a Libertarian view of freedoms where governments should assume maximal liberty of each couple and only restrict a liberty to prevent a clear and obvious harm to someone else from the exercise of that liberty. But the "Anything Goes" school of experimentation has risks, too, and should be tempered with evidence about safety and benefits.

As said, bioconservativism is at bottom a religious view, and a dark one at that. Why? Well, we can't believe that we are "fallen" unless we had some place to "fall" from. Arguments that emphasize that scientists and humans lack the wisdom to attempt enhancement assume the Fall of Man and Original Sin.

I have said that bioconservatism is religious or semi-religious, but of a certain kind, namely, pessimistic religion. Pessimistic religion always endorses the status quo; it always opposes medical innovation as unnatural. Pessimistic religion fears change in medicine, the most famous example of which is anesthesia in childbirth: "In sorrow thou shalt bring forth children" (Genesis 3:16). So ministers thundered against painless birth until Queen Victoria silenced them with her demand for relief, setting an example for millions of other women, who embraced a more positive view of what religion required.

Indeed, one wonders whether modern religion can ever affirm new options in medicine. Here's a doctoral thesis for a young theology student interested in bioethics: Can modern religions have a voice other than, as Nietzsche said, "Nay-Saying" in bioethics? As Alasdair MacIntyre might say, what medical advances is religion *for?*

It's not enough for religions to position themselves as the brakes on the runaway train of medical change. Progress in medicine always needs support. Controversial innovations don't become "change" or "progress" unless they enlist enough patients, families, and physicians to support them.

Instead of a runaway train, medical progress is more like pulling a heavily loaded freight train uphill where toll collectors every hundred yards demand fees while querying why the train needs to go further.

In retrospect, and *from the start*, religion should have gotten behind assisted reproduction, rather than opposing it tooth and nail. What can be more pro-life and pro-family than helping infertile couples create their own babies?

Some would object to my equation of religion in bioethics to the reactionary views of Leon Kass, Daniel Callahan, and the Vatican. Many theists today reject the premise of the fallen nature of humans and the conception of a primitive, vindictive God who would create humans with a nature that inherently tends to sin. Instead, modern theologians posit a more loving God who created free, compassionate beings capable of reflection, growth, and understanding.

But when theologians confront change in bioethics, they usually revert to being bioconservatives, checking in at the old Fallen Hotel, taking a room among their Alarmist brethren. That is the comfortable way of doing bioethics among clergy: to prohibit, to urge caution, to warn, and to urge complete consensus on a committee where one skeptic can prevent agreement.

Of course, transhumanists can be equally selective in the descriptions they advance. They may describe the successful enhancements that occurred in dentistry (from saving bad teeth to improving appearance), in optometry (from eyeglasses to laser surgery), in public health (from public sanitation to vaccinations), and medicine (from antibiotics to high-tech emergency response systems). In these accounts, they may overlook the many false starts, the many victims of experimentation, and the undemocratic nature of the decisions that created many of these advances.

As said, Enthusiasm promoted gene therapy and genetic enhancement with breathless hype. It ignored the complexities of gene-gene interactions with complex environments, as well as the ethical difficulties of determining which packages of causes create which traits. It also ignored problems of vaccinations in the history of that field.

But Alarmism has ruled for too many years, indeed too many decades, and if we must choose between frames, maybe it's time for a little Enthusiasm. Increases in longevity and new tools from stem cells could reveal new vistas for humans, if only we possess the will to go forward. I shall argue that we can do so, and do so *ethically*.

■■■

This brief history of bioethics over the last half-century has two lessons, each learned painfully: treat different kinds of cases differently and be aware of the simplistic frame inside which we tell most stories in bioethics. Real life and good ethical analysis are, and should be, more complex, and will be treated as such if we just look at real cases.

NOTES

1. After a new hearing where three new people testified about her wishes, physicians removed Nancy's feeding tube. With so many witnesses in agreement, the Cruzans met the clear-and-convincing standard and the feeding tube was removed.

2. President's Council on Bioethics, "Better Children," Chapter 2, *Beyond Therapy: Biotechnology and the Pursuit of Happiness* (Washington, D.C.: Dana Press, 2003), 30–45.

3. Walter Kornberg, *Science News*, 1969.

4. John Evans, *Playing God: Human Genetic Engineering and the Rationalization of Public Debate* (Chicago: University of Chicago Press, 2002).

5. June Goodfield, *Playing God: Genetic Engineering and the Manipulation of Life* (New York: Random House, 1977).

6. Jeremy Rifkin and Ted Howard, *Who Should Play God? : The artificial creation of life and what it means for the future of the human race,* (New York: Delacorte, 1977).

7. Rollin Hotchkiss, quoted by Ronald Kotulak, "And Now Your Child Built to Order: Day of Genetic Engineer Near, Biologist Says," *Chicago Tribune*, August 18, 1965, 5.

8. F. M. Burnett , quoted by Howard Simons, "Genetic Defect Victims Are Urged Not to Wed," *Washington Post*, April 26, 1966, A1.

9. James Shannon, quoted by Howard Simons, "Genetic Defect Victims Are Urged Not to Wed," *Washington Post*, April 26, 1966, A10.

10. Francis Galton, *Hereditary Genius* (London: MacMillan, 1869); J. B. S. Haldane, *Deadalus* (1924); James Watson, quoted in Michael Gerson, "The Eugenics Temptation," *Washington Post,* October 24, 2007.

11. Gregory Stock, *Redesigning Humans: Our Inevitable Genetic Future* (New York: Houghton Mifflin, 2002).

12. James Hughes, *Citizen Cyborg* (New York: Basic Books, 2004); Ramez Naam, *More Than Human: Embracing the Promise of Biological Enhancement* (New York: Broadway, 2005)

Chapter Three

Expanding the Mind

In preparing for law boards, Tiffany struggles to master huge amounts of material while teaching biology in high school. She hopes to pass and join a law firm. For a week before the exam, she takes modafinil, obtained legally from a sympathetic psychiatrist. Like Eddie Morra in *Limitless,* on modafinil Tiffany feels she can master anything and ace her exams ("a tablet a day and I was limitless," says Eddie). Tiffany takes the exam on modafinil, but crashes afterward and misses two days at school. But with the aide of modafinil, Tiffany passes with a high score.

Did Tiffany do anything wrong? Dangerous? Risk becoming dependent on modafinil for success in stressful situations? Did she cheat when she took her exam on a drug that others had not taken?

Before answering those questions, consider the drugs people now take toward the same goal. Caffeine is currently the world's most popular cognitive enhancer. If we include the caffeine in coffee, tea, cocoa, soft drinks, and energy drinks, billions of people every day ingest cognitive enhancers. Nicotine also stimulates the brain. French writers from Balzac to Sartre wrote while drinking pots of coffee and smoking packs of cigarettes.

If we could study enhancers in a calm, scientific way, we might discover better cognitively enhancing drugs. Although the effects fade over hours, caffeine is an addictive drug and desire for it builds over time. When people accustomed to several cups of coffee a day quit, they experience headaches and withdrawal. Although caffeine has proved to be remarkably safe, it also stimulates the heart, so we need a more selective enhancer, the way cyclosporine selectively inhibits rejection of transplanted organs. And of course, nicotine is customarily taken in products that damage the lungs and thus cause cancer, so people need a substitute for it.

Modafinil is known more commonly by its first trademarked name, Provigil. Not an amphetamine, modafinil stimulates wakefulness and allows its users to get the same effect on four hours as on eight hours of regular sleep. Originally created by a French company to treat narcolepsy, modafinil has been used in the last decade to fight chronic fatigue syndrome. Physicians also prescribe it for sleep-shift workers, soldiers who need to stay vigilant on long missions, sleep apnea, and for the "brain fog" that often accompanies chemotherapy or coronary bypass surgery.

Modafinil is not harmless and has not been tested in large general populations. In heavy dosages, modafinil causes dermatological problems such as acne and eczema. It suppresses appetite, causes insomnia, headache, nausea, nervousness, and hypertension. It increases wakefulness and it may increase ability to focus.

The FDA approved Provigil for Cephalon in 1998. Nearly a decade later in 2006, Cephalon tried to get Provigil approved under the name of Sparlon to treat Attention Deficit and Hypersensitivity Disorder. However, the medical committee advising the FDA discovered that some patients using modafinil developed severe skin rashes. Concerned that Sparlon might be marketed to far more adults than Provigil, even adolescents and children, the committee voted twelve-to-one against it.

Scientists do not know exactly how modafinil works, and the fact that it is not thoroughly studied or understood should warn us about its potential dangers. After all, cocaine and amphetamines were once thought to be neither dangerous nor addictive.

Amphetamines stimulate everything in the central nervous system, including the heart rate, whereas modafinil selectively stimulates wakefulness without causing hyper-alertness, heart palpations, or nervousness. Modafinil increases histamines in the hypothalamus and the release of neurotransmitters called monoamines.

The FDA has monitored modafinil's usage for over a decade, and it requires that physicians report all adverse events from such usage, which includes suicides, skin reactions, and other harms. So far, few such events have been reported. At this inchoate stage, it may not be addictive like amphetamines (although at least two researchers disagree[1]). Thus, use of modafinil may be physically safe for competent adults. As said, there have been no systematic studies of its widespread usage over decades.

The FDA approves a new drug for one purpose—the official one on the drug's label—and then physicians informally may test it for other purposes by prescribing it "off label." It is not clear how often physicians report adverse side effects of off-label drug usage, so this could mean more people have problems than have been reported.

All this seems less revolutionary when we realize that large amounts of caffeine may create alertness just as effectively as modafinil. In fact, caffeine is a more potent cognitive enhancer than many people realize, and people may take far more of it than they admit.

The Center for Science and the Public Interest says that a 16-ounce (Grande) serving of Starbucks coffee contains 320 milligrams of caffeine. In contrast, a 12-ounce can of Jolt Cola contains 72 milligrams of caffeine; Diet Coke contains 47 milligrams of caffeine.[2]

Consider this interesting fact about caffeine. In groundbreaking research, Li-Huei Tsai of MIT developed a quick way to mimic Alzheimer's-like symptoms in mice and an innovative method to test memory in these mice. According to the *NOVA* show that featured Tsai's benchmark-to-bedside research, another study found that *giving the same kind of mice the equivalent of five cups of coffee a day for two months allowed them to recover the same memories.*[3]

Maybe caffeine is already as good as modafinil for helping the brain. Like aspirin, it may be more efficacious than scientists realize. If aspirin and caffeine had not been discovered, either today as new patented drugs would make billions for pharmacological companies. Use of both has been proven effective and safe.

Given the data indicating safety, should competent adults such as Tiffany be allowed to take modafinil not for any quasi-medical dysfunction but simply to increase her performance? Let's suppose it's easy for Tiffany to get a prescription for modafinil, no harder than it is now to get one for a tranquilizer such as lorazepam, an antidepressant such as flouoxetine, or for the five million who take them, Ritalin or Adderal. Even if they must see a physician every month for monitoring, many people find these drugs easy to get.

This is not one of those notorious desert island cases of some philosophers. A 2008 online survey of the journal *Nature* revealed that an astonishing 20 percent of readers had already taken one of three legal drugs to enhance their mental abilities (methylphenidate, modafinil, and beta blockers, e.g., atenolol).[4] Donepezil, marketed under one trademark as Aricept, prevents the decline of memory in patients with early stages of Alzheimer's disease. Some researchers think the same drug used on the same neural pathways, which increases concentration of the neurotransmitter acetylcholine, will increase memory in healthy people, and take donepezil to enhance their brains.

Whether it's modafinil or Virtual Life, the key philosophical question becomes: *Is it intrinsically wrong to use these mental enhancers?*

To emphasize what kind of question I am asking, notice that using cognitive enhancers could be *indirectly wrong* because of many reasons: they might not work, making them a waste of money; they might have dangerous effects that we might not know for many years (modafinil might cause brain tumors); they might lead to greater inequality; in using them, we might lose something important in society; using them might later harm others; or their use might send the wrong message to disadvantaged groups.

But I am not here asking any of those questions. Instead, I am asking whether it could be *just wrong* to employ cognitive enhancement. In other words, is it *morally forbidden* to try to change my self, my memory, and my brain? Is changing myself this way wrong in itself, something I have no right to do? Am I obligated not to do this? Am I an evil person if I try to grow my mind, not through education or meditation, but biochemically, or with machines, or by escaping this world? If I'm successful, am I a freak?

Suppose Hannah takes modafinil to increase her performance to do the *New York Times* crossword puzzles, puzzles that grow harder as the week progresses. At the end of the week, if Hannah has worked all the puzzles for the first time in her life, should she be elated? Critics would say that modafinil, not her authentic self, worked the puzzles. But Balzac wrote his great novels using caffeine and nicotine, so are his works suspect? Admirers would say that modafinil *focused* the resources of Hannah's and Balzac's brains, allowing them to function maximally.

Nevertheless, naturalistic intuitions nag us that Hannah cheated. If she can't finish the puzzle "herself" and can only do so on a drug, has "she" really finished it?

John Stuart Mill in *On Liberty* wrote:

The only part of conduct of any one, for which he is amenable to society, is that which concerns others. In the part, which merely concerns himself, his independence is, of right, absolute. Over himself, over his *own body and mind*, the individual is sovereign.[5] (emphasis added)

On Mill's view, my enhancement of my mental life could only be wrong, could only be a moral issue, if it threatens harm to others.

Such harms may exist, and we will examine them soon, but suppose we ask the solitary question of a financially secure, single adult with no responsibilities to children or aged parents, just an atomistic individual wishing to experience greater cognitive powers. So now we can ask the question in its purest form: is it intrinsically wrong for her to try to enhance her mental powers?

Enthusiasts can see no reason why it is. Just as it is not intrinsically wrong to work long hours by taking lots of caffeinated products, or to use the Internet all day at work in trading stocks, or to retreat after work into Virtual Life, nothing about better versions of these drugs, machines, or fantasies justifies calling them intrinsically wrong.

Indeed, Mill would put the onus of proof on any group or government that would limit a person's freedom to change oneself. Why should there be any limits at all on what a person can do to improve his or her mind?

Bioconservative Alarmists argue that I do not have the right to change my brain because its special value comes from its uniqueness, from its being given to me by God and not manufactured, from its being natural, and from its being fundamental to who I am. In enhancing my brain, I risk changing my identity, and I should not do that.

Even if that's true, isn't it up to me to risk changes to my identity? For most kids, going off to West Point or to a big sports-obsessed, fraternity-dominated university risks a change of identity, but can't people make that decision?

Going back to factors that enhance thinking, neuroscientist, Enthusiast, and dissenting member of the President's Council on Bioethics Michael Gazzinga argued, "What is the difference between Ritalin and the Kaplan SAT review? It's six of one and a half dozen of the other. If both can boost SAT scores by, say, 120 points, I think it's immaterial which way it's done."[6]

Alarmists object that mental enhancement is to gain an edge, not to fend off death. But let us take that objection, give it some rope, and see if it hangs itself. Now, of course, we are sidestepping the view that using enhancements is intrinsically wrong, and moving to indirect arguments.

In most walks of life—academia, finance, law, engineering, medicine, and computers—losing mental acuity is a kind of death. When the command goes, so goes the whole system. Consider the most plausible ethical situation where competent adults merely wish to *maintain* their normal mental functioning. Who can argue against, say, a tax accountant's wish to continue providing for his family? If the stock market takes a dive and retirement accounts are wiped out, who would deprive similar professionals from working longer in order to accumulate adequate monies?

"Yes, but!" Alarmists retort, if you open that gate, too much goes through. To allow competent accountants to maintain maximal mental functioning into their eighties will also allow thirty-year-olds to *improve* their functioning. Patients in their thirties will claim they need the same enhancers to get a job and care for an aging parent, to compete in the world market, and so on. It will be a reverse slippery slope, with a tidal wave surging upward, pressuring everyone to take cognitive enhancers.

Well, that's partly true, although not all baseball players take steroids. Moreover, Enthusiasts retort, this objection ignores the likelihood that productivity, creativity, and pleasure could also increase dramatically. Few people would enter a time machine and return to a time when they couldn't use the Internet to find medical information or use a phone to call friends. If tens of millions could safely use modafinil, who knows what new knowledge might be discovered, what new music created, what new theorems proved?

Nevertheless, perhaps the benefits to the general public would not be as great as Enthusiasts hope. Studies to date of the benefits of modafinil suggest small benefits and are limited to small studies of a few people. It could be that the smartest, most creative people get the most benefit, or the dullest, but not average people. Compared to the brain-boosting effects of computers and caffeine, the extra boost from modafinil might be small. It's not going to change Forrest Gump into Einstein.

However, Alarmists have another trump card in their hand here. As in the first chapter, the unmentioned elephant in the room in this discussion is addiction. *Addiction* should be distinguished from *dependence*. Addiction is biochemical, where because of increased tolerance to the drug, users need more and more of the same substance to achieve the same effect. Dependence is psychological, becoming habituated to using the drug to perform a task and feeling incompetent to do it without it.

New research suggests that the thrill of certain kinds of experience releases dopamine in the brain, which produces a kind of feedback loop much like that caused by opium or cocaine.[7] Thus, wins in gambling or sexual conquests release chemicals that could be just as addictive as alcohol, caffeine, or heroin.

An important issue about addiction to mind-enhancing chemicals is the Exposure Effect. If you legalize the sale of alcohol in a previously dry county, a percentage of that county's previously teetotaling citizens will become heavy drinkers or alcoholics. Ditto with gambling.

Alarmists correctly predict that with greater exposure to the Internet, smart phones, Starbucks coffee, or modafinil, more people will become dependent/addicted on these cognitive enhancers. This is both because people like acting smarter and because biochemical changes take place with the rush of mental victories.

Alarmists emphasize that the dangers of addiction to new brain enhancers are real. At Princeton's Institute for Advanced Study, the Hungarian Paul Erdös, one of the most gifted and prolific mathematicians of the twentieth century, abused amphetamines, but used them to prove many theorems in mathematics. According to one biography of Erdös, to win a bet that he could not, Erdös once gave up amphetamines for a month. When asked if it had been worth it, he replied that during his abstinence, mathematics had been set back a month: "Before, when I looked at a piece of blank paper my mind was filled with ideas. Now all I see is a blank piece of paper."[8] After he won the bet, he resumed using amphetamines. (He influenced mathematics so much that his friends, students, and followers assign themselves "Erdös numbers" to boast how much he directly taught them, with a "1" as the highest number.)

Does Erdös's use of amphetamines devalue that achievement? Although such usage makes him a poor role model for teenage math prodigies, a proof is still a proof. However, the same mental powers involved in making proofs may have also given Erdös resistance to other dangers of amphetamine addiction. Also, as a Fellow of the Institute for Advanced Studies, he didn't need to worry about money and thus, about paying for his addiction—an unusual circumstance. Professional poker player Paul Phillips claimed that the use of modafinil and methylphenidate made him better and helped him earn $2.3 million playing poker. "The drugs improved my concentration during high-stakes tournaments," he said, allowing him to better track all the action at his table.[9]

In a prequel to *Limitless*, *Slate* writer David Plotz planned to take 100 milligrams of modafinil for a week as an experiment and see how productive it made him and whether he slept well on it. To write on deadline, he took modafinil in the morning, felt like Superman for fifteen hours and did not want to go to sleep, but did anyway, woke up refreshed, worked another great fifteen-hour-day, but then, fearing he would become addicted, panicked, quit, and did not take it again.[10]

But let's not downplay the damage of drug addiction, especially to mind-enhancing drugs. By 2000, an epidemic of addiction to methamphetamines had swept rural America and parts of the world, alerting us to the dangers of this drug. From the epidemic of abuse of amphetamines in rural America and Mexico, we've learned the hard way about the exposure effect. Even if only 2 percent of users in the general population became addicted to modafinil, that's millions of harmed people.

Minnesota had so many convicts with "Dew mouth"—no teeth from excessive consumption of Mountain Dew and from grinding teeth due to agitation on methamphetamine—that whether to provide them with false teeth became an ethical issue of allocation of its limited state resources.[11] Many states have now taken steps to restrict sales of cold medicines containing ephedrine and pseudoephedrine, ingredients needed to make methamphetamine.

But modafinil is not an amphetamine, Enthusiasts retort. Indeed, it seems more like caffeine than amphetamine. Enthusiasts again pose a key ethical question: should we allow adults to use modafinil when many users might become dependent on it?

One compromise between Enthusiasm and Alarmism is to continue the present arrangement, allowing modafinil by prescription, and hence allowing it to be monitored, but not banned. This makes physicians gatekeepers of such drugs and decision makers about therapy, enhancement, and whether that distinction has moral relevance. Also, if modafinil turns out to be addictive and not just to cause dependence, then physicians could restrict prescriptions, or the FDA could declare modafinil a Class-III drug, subject to more careful monitoring. This does not completely answer the question in public policy, which queries how common such prescriptions should be. Do we want to go down the road of Ritalin and Adderall, which five million American children now take? Or antidepressants such as Prozac and Zoloft, which another six million Americans take? In 2020, do we want four million American managers and professionals on modafinil?

Well, assume the big numbers, and assume that four million American adults do want to work on modafinil. Is that number in itself a *reductio ad absurdum* of expanded availability?

Yes, Enthusiasts argue, some harm will ensue, but so will enormous benefits, including satisfactions perhaps undreamed of by current thinkers. Although a small percentage of a normal population will become dependent, most people will handle modafinil, outgrow it, or choose to forego it when taking it conflicts with other values. That means that a cost-benefit judgment must be made between the good of increased mental performance by say, 98 percent of people, and the impairment of the addicted 2 percent.

Personally, I worry about something that neither Alarmists nor Enthusiasts commonly discuss. I worry that drug companies will push modafinil and its clones on people in hopes of creating golden cash cows—if modafinil could increase cognitive performance and retain its results, Big Pharma could make billions. But my hunch is that if it could produce such results, millions of people would be using modafinil now, the way people take anabolic steroids to build muscle mass and find physicians to write them prescriptions, and drug companies would be covertly promoting modafinil's usage. The problem is that we don't know, but my hunch is that modafinil will not have the same results in everyone, will not be that superior to caffeine, and will not help memory, but only focus.

If modafinil worked well, then I believe we would have an arms race and more and more productive people would need to take it. After all, if every other professor, physician, writer, lawyer, or engineer takes it and performs better than I, what choice do I really have? If I want to succeed, I must perform at the norm of my group.

Like Virtual Life and a fantasy life divorced from reality, the decision to take modafinil should be a personal one, but that does not mean we cannot rationally evaluate personal values. Personally, if I could only write books or papers on modafinil, I would worry that something is wrong with me. "Why can't I just write on coffee?" I would ask. If I were Tiffany, I would have a nagging doubt that I could not have passed the Law Boards on my own, and that doubt might grow, making me less confident that I could do any big, intense project on my own. Such worries might make me hoard modafinil, lest my supply of the drug ever became interrupted.

And if Tiffany, or four million professors, became dependent on modafinil, what would happen if the supply did cease? If the FDA discovered it caused atrophy of the brain and revoked it? Or the pharmaceutical company, realizing people's dependence, doubled, then quadrupled its price? What if it became so expensive, or illegal, that people began doing wrong things to get it?

As a personal value, you can't start taking any drug with addictive potential with "eyes wide shut." You must evaluate your own potential for addiction, whatever the potentially addicting substance or activity is. For me, coffee is enough.

NOTES

1. "Addictive Qualities of Modafinil Not Discussed by FDA Advisory," Alliance for Human Research Protection, March 28, 2006. http://www.ahr org/cms/content/view/130/28/
2. Center for Science and the Public Interest, "Caffeine Content of Food & Drugs," 2007. http://www.cspinet.org/new/cafchart.htm
3. "Science Now: Of Mice and Memory," NOVA, Corporation for Public Broadcasting, June 25, 2008. http://www.pbs.org/wgbh/nova/sciencenow/0301/bios.html
4. "Some Professors Pop Pills for an Intellectual Edge," *Chronicle of Higher Education*, April 25, 2008, A1.
5. John Stuart Mill, *On Liberty*, 1869 (many editions).
6. James Hughes, *Citizen Cyborg*, 37.
7. Trevor W. Robbins and Barry J. Everitt, "Drug Addiction: Bad Habits Add Up," *NATURE*, 398, no.15, (April, 1999).www.nature.com
8. "Paul Erdös," Wikipedia, quoting from J. Hill's *Paul Erdös: Mathematical Genius, Human (In That Order)*.
9. Karen Kaplan and Denise Joshe, "Academics, Musicians, Even Poker Champs Use Pills to Sharpen their Minds, Legally," *Los Angeles Times*, December 20, 2007.
10. David Plotz, "Wake Up, Little Susie: Can We Sleep Less?" *Slate,* March 7, 2003.http://www.slate.com/id/2079113/

11. "Mobile Clinic Treats 'Mountain Dew Mouth'," ABC News 20/20, February 13, 2009; "What is Mountain Dew Mouth?" *WiseGeek*, http://www.wisegeek.com/what-is-mountain-dew-mouth.htm

Chapter Four

Building Better Female Bodies

Jennifer is a thirty-two-year-old single competent female who has transformed her body over the last decade, from a stick-like Plain Jane to a voluptuous Valkyrie. She has had liposuction, breast implants, facial surgery, and to refine her new body, used drugs, exercise, and diet. While previously hating her body, she now displays it by wearing revealing outfits. When people glance at her, she basks in their attention.

Is there anything wrong with Jennifer? With what thousands of other women like her want to do? If something has gone bad with Jennifer, is it a moral matter or just one of different personal values? Is what Jennifer has done enhancement or disfigurement? How do we know the difference? Should society encourage or discourage such changes?

For some philosophers, what Jennifer has done is not a moral issue and cannot be. After all, it's her body, her life, and what she does with it has little chance of harming others.

Alas, as a century of scholarship on *On Liberty* has taught us, the distinction between self-regarding and other-regarding actions is not a sharp one. If some women start to enlarge their breasts or have face-lifts, it affects the norm and how other women feel about their bodies. What appears to be a purely personal issue in enhancement ethics may not be. Indeed, the range of the merely personal is itself an ethical issue in this debate.

The ethics of changing the human body has a pedigree. The ancient Greeks sought beauty in perfectly sculpted bodies to match the bodies of their gods. In the 1300s, Chinese bound the feet of little girls to make them tiny and lady-like.[1] Renaissance women strove for blondish-red hair, proportionately delicate bodies, and light-complexioned skin.[2] By stretching the necks of girls with bands of metal, some African and Asian cultures tried to create long, graceful necks.[3]

Philosophers Margaret Olivia Little and Susan Bordo believe that current female norms of appearance reflect social constructions and that cosmetic surgery unethically reinforces such norms.[4] They criticize the values of individuals who choose cosmetic surgery, the physicians who offer it, and the society that reinforces it.

Professor Little calls this serious objection "complicity with suspect norms." She argues that the proper end of medicine should not be in helping women reshape their bodies to look like Barbie dolls. Others, such as physician-bioethicist Howard Brody and bioethicist Frank Miller, argue that physicians who offer such surgery violate the internal norms of medicine and its ideal of compassionate therapy.[5] They argue that cosmetic surgery is not what medicine should be *for*.

Social norms direct cosmetic surgery differently for distinct ethnic groups. For example, the most popular surgery among Asian women is double eyelid surgery, in which surgeons create a crease in the eyelid, whose effect is to make a bigger, rounder, more Western eye. Critics dislike how surgeons are altering Asian bodies to fit Western ideals. "You want to be part of the acceptable culture and the acceptable ethnicity, so you want to look more Westernized," said Margaret M. Chin, a professor of sociology at Hunter College who specializes in Asian immigrant culture. "I feel sad that they feel like they have to do this."[6] About 5 percent of Asians have some form of cosmetic surgery, about 750,000 in 2009 and about double the number in 2000 (versus 4 percent of Caucasians and 3 percent of Latinos).

One perspective on what Jennifer has done is that she is *cheating*. Why? She is pretending to be someone she is not. She is presenting herself to others, to men, in a body that is not her natural body. Isn't that cheating those who interact with her? I'll return to this issue later.

Another important issue about the ethics of enhancement concerns money. In bioethics, to understand an issue, always consider the money. You do not have to be a Marxist to appreciate the insight that how people make money influences their views. So if surgeons make money performing surgery, Marx would predict that—all other things being equal—surgeons would urge clients to have more surgery rather than less.

In the current scheme of medical reimbursement, something about money cries out about enhancement. Because insurance companies do not reimburse physicians for it, physicians doing this kind of medicine get paid directly by clients. Patient autonomy combines with consumer sovereignty to push medicine past its old boundaries.

Clients pay surgeons and dermatologists directly for weekly botox injections or for breast surgery. To do so, clients take out loans or make monthly payments over years on a schedule set up by the physician's office. This is far from the image of the compassionate country doctor accepting a chicken as payment from the poor patient.

These facts about money alter the moral landscape, and it is strange that so few discussions to date of the ethics of medical enhancement have analyzed how it does. It explains in part why so many people undergo too many cosmetic procedures too many times, too early, and in inappropriate circumstances.

One might argue that direct compensation doesn't differ that much to the physician from compensation from insurance companies: either way, the more she operates, the more she makes. But that is not correct, for insurance companies have medical review by physicians and try not to pay for inappropriate surgery. But a rich woman may pay for several facelifts and be subject to only the review of her surgeon, who may praise the way she looks, even if she looks terrible.

An irony exists here, similar to one about assisted reproduction. For reasons connected to research on live-born fetuses, Congress in the mid-1970s banned federal funding of any experiment using human embryos or fetuses. Most insurance companies followed suit and did not pay for in vitro fertilization. When couples paid for such services with their own money, and clinics financed their own research from such payments, they realized that this financial cloud had an unexpected silver lining: they were not subject to review by the National Institutes of Health, local Institutional Review Boards, or committees at insurance companies doing medical review. In short, and much to the subsequent dismay of critics, they could do whatever kind of research they wanted.

Much the same thing has happened with cosmetic medicine. Although some techniques grew out of ordinary medicine—breast augmentation grew out of techniques for breast reconstruction after mastectomies—surgeons developed many techniques exclusively for enhancement and financed those developments from patients' fees. As such, most physicians who offer enhancement advertise for services as if they were selling cars. And like car salesmen, who are not out to sell you the best car for the least amount of money, so some physicians don't sell clients the least amount of enhancement they need.

Worse, some patients don't know where to stop. If someone has been through weeks of swelling from cosmetic surgery on her face, and believes she looks much better, and has paid $10,000, it is difficult for the surgeon to tell her that she looks worse.

A related topic about the ethics of physicians in enhancement medicine concerns the outer boundaries of medicine. Now two types of physicians constantly push those boundaries: those in clinical research and those in assisted reproduction. It is inevitable that traditional physicians will find distasteful some procedures done by physicians in enhancement medicine, just as they find distasteful techniques of assisted reproduction. It is also true that malpractice is typically defined in state law as departing from the "customary and normal procedures of the medical community."

Some critics worry that money paid for enhancement is diverted from other areas where it could be used better. But this is a specious argument: if I choose to buy an expensive car, forbidding me to do so does not entail that I will give the same money for relief of famine. Preventing physicians from entering enhancement medicine does not mean they will become physicians in primary care. It doesn't work that way, just as preventing women from enlarging their breasts doesn't mean the nonspent money will be diverted to better prenatal care for poor women.

What is true is that one part of medicine may distort the whole. If cash fuels one part of medicine, and the rest sags under paperwork and regulation, young, restless physicians will gravitate to the easier, flashier parts. And if huge distortions occur, national public policy must correct the imbalance.

So now we know that physical enhancement may serve dubious norms and those providing it may have conflicts of interest in giving impartial advice to clients about safety and risks. So what are the risks?

In North America and across the world during the last decades, surgical and pharmacological enhancement of the body has exploded. Between 2000 and 2007, 50,000 Norwegian women had breast implants.[7] Such surgeries carry risk. Much cosmetic surgery is performed in outpatient, nonhospital settings. Florida has the best data on incidents in such settings because of its mandatory reporting law, having seven years of good data covering March 2000 to March 2007.[8] In these years, 31 patients died and 143 had serious complications, about 60 percent of which occurred after aesthetic surgeries. Liposuction under general anesthesia caused a significant number of these deaths.

Surgeons during the last decades performed vast numbers of cosmetic surgeries, and the most popular procedures were lipoplasty (liposuction), breast enlargement, breast reduction, rhinoplasty (nose jobs), eyelid surgery, facelifts, and botox injections.[9] Such surgery carries more risks than is commonly portrayed on television shows. Eight percent of French plastic surgeons have experienced a case of deep vein thrombosis and over half have had a patient with a pulmonary embolism.[10]

Consider bariatric surgery, considered by some to be a frivolous shortcut by obese people to normal weight. Such surgery can be a medical treatment of last resort when obesity threatens life. Morbid obesity causes diabetes, heart failure, breathing problems, bone breakage, passivity, and arthritis. A normal person's Body Mass Index (BMI) varies between 18 and 25. A BMI of 25 to 30 classifies a person as medically obese; one over 30, as "morbidly obese." The latter shortens lives dramatically.

According to the American Society of Bariatric Surgery Web site, bariatric surgery increased from 37,000 surgeries in 2000 to 177,000 surgeries in 2006.[11] Obviously, the same surgical techniques that extend lives of morbidly obese people also remove fat from arms, legs, stomach, and hips of less obese people, and thus, can enhance normality. But bariatric surgery carries significant risks and should not be considered as a quick, safe way to lose weight.

Liposuction is the most frequently performed cosmetic operation in Germany. Because of a liberal reimbursement system, between 1998 and 2003 German physicians did about 250,000 liposuctions, giving them good data from which to estimate risks.[12]

In those years of liposuctions, twenty-three patients died and about fifty others had extremely serious complications, such as necrotizing faciitis, gas gangrene, and sepsis. Almost as severe, other patients suffered pulmonary embolisms, hemorrhages, and perforation of internal abdominal organs. Lack of surgical experience and selection of unfit patients caused these problems, as well as unsterile techniques, which, in modern times, is unforgivable.

"Body contouring" with liposuction, even if safe, does not always achieve pleasing results. Physicians sometimes do not remove enough fat, leave palpable and visible irregularities, suck out too much fat, and the surgery itself generally creates hematomas, infections, swelling and bruising.[13]

Perhaps the most suspicious facial enhancement is botox injections. Botox is a neural toxin originating from *Clostridium botulinum*, which causes deadly botulism in meat. In moderate dosages, botox can be highly poisonous to humans. Some critics suggest that, over years, botox injections can leach into the brain.[14]

As therapy, botox can treat female urinary incontinence.[15] By paralyzing the muscles that urge women to urinate, researchers help such women gain more control over their bladders. Botox blocks neurotransmission in muscles, so as therapy, it's also used to treat facial tics in adults or uncontrollable, muscular spasms in children.

For improving the youthful look of faces, doctors inject tiny amounts of botox to paralyze the facial muscles that create wrinkles. To maintain this effect, clients must see doctors every few months at a cost of $100-$200 per treatment. Botox creates a constant river of money for physicians who inject it because, to maintain the look, patients must get re-injected every few months *as long as they live*. (As one plastic surgeon says, "The amount of money you can make and the amount of time you spend [giving Botox] is unparalleled. You can make as much money Botoxing someone's face in ten minutes as you can do in a two- or three-hour operation."[16]

Facelifts are risky. Its most common complications (15 percent of cases) are hematomas, localized swelling filled with blood.[17] Facelifts in the twentieth century displayed overly tight skin or, when things really went wrong, a "Joker line" from a corner of a mouth to a cheek.[18] A prominent Manhattan plastic surgeon derides such antiquated results, claiming that the proper way to do this operation now is to leave patients with the flexible, bouncy skin of youngsters, not the tautly stretched, mummified look of old facelifts.[19]

Surgeons developed breast reconstruction with silicone gels to help women after mastectomies and later used these techniques to augment or decrease breasts for healthy women. In the 1950s and 1960s, surgeons used crude methods to augment breasts of 50,000 women, such as directly injecting silicone into them. In some cases, the tissue around the silicone became inflamed, hardened, and painful, so surgeons had to later perform mastectomies to remove everything. This is now considered a bad practice.

In the early 1960s, surgeons began implanting silicone-filled rubber bags, either between the chest wall and the pectoral muscles or between pectoral muscles and the breast. Dow Corning manufactured these bags. A decade later, surgeons used a less viscous silicone gel and a thinner sac, resulting in more ruptures. Claiming they had been harmed, women in the 1970s began class-action lawsuits against Dow Corning.

Because of these lawsuits, surgeons started to use saline-filled bags. However, even this procedure led to major complications including capsular contractures, when the rubber sac tightens and squeezes the saline, causing leakage from the capsule.

After three decades of silicone implants, over 400,000 women registered in 1995 as potential claimants in nearly 20,000 lawsuits against Dow Corning.[20] That May, because of costs of defending itself against these lawsuits, Dow Corning filed for Chapter 11 bankruptcy. In 1998, it filed for bankruptcy reorganization; to settle all claims against it, it agreed to compensate women for removal of breast implants or ruptures of silicone in them.

All the class-action suits in federal courts came to a head under the late federal judge Sam C. Pointer in Birmingham, AL., who in 1998 appointed four independent experts to review claims that the implants harmed women. These court-appointed masters concluded that medical evidence did not show that the implants caused any serious diseases. In 1999, the Institute of Medicine concluded the same, stating that although implants caused local scarring and hardening of surrounding tissues, they did not cause serious disease.[21] Several other large studies around the world came to the same conclusion.

At the end of 2011, about 70,000 women in France, Brazil, and Venezuela were told that they had received implants with an inferior, industrial-grade silicone rather than surgical silicone.[22] The latter is less likely to leak and, if it does, to cause irritation and inflammation. France offered to pay for its 30,000 women to undergo "explants."[23]

Even if breast implants don't cause disease, some women didn't know enough before they got them. In one survey in 2007, 40 percent of women with implants believed that, before they had their surgeries, they should have learned more about their complications.[24] Perhaps they did not have the "serious disease" investigated by Judge Pointer and the Institute of Medicine, but thirty years later, some women reported neurological and rheumatological problems. In one study of a hundred women who had their implants removed, rheumatologists diagnosed autoimmune or rheumatic disease in eighteen of them. In this class of women, 75 percent had lost some sensitivity in their nipples, and twenty-five patients had lost all sensation.[25] These women had 186 implants removed, and of these, 57 percent had failed by rupturing or leaking, and bacteria infected 42 percent.

All implants eventually need to be replaced. Even with the best, third-generation implants, after ten years, 15 percent of women have implants replaced.[26] As one cosmetic surgeon says, "A lot of people have the wrong idea about augmentations. They don't know that implants are not a lifetime device and that you're going to have to have them replaced. If you have them at twenty, you're probably going to have four or five revision surgeries over the course of your life."[27]

Did most women who had implants years ago get informed consent about this? Did they know that women who smoke have twice the rate of complications as nonsmokers?[28] That for women getting experimental or premarket implants at discounted fees, after three years, the rate of reoperations runs as high as 20 percent?[29]

The proliferation of specialty boards confuses patients, even those who only want to use a "board-certified" physician. The American Society of Plastic Surgeons certifies almost all (90 percent) of America's plastic surgeons. Another organization, the American Society for Aesthetic Plastic Surgery, also certifies plastic surgeons, but this society may have been formed in part by those who could not get, or refused to try to get, certified by the ASPS.

Contrary to what most people believe, any physician can do cosmetic surgery. A physician does not need to do a residency in cosmetic surgery to operate cosmetically. Dermatologists may operate cosmetically, and most who do belong to the American Society for Dermatologic Surgery. In some states, *dentists* can legally perform any surgery above the neck.

With the growing popularity of cosmetic surgery and lack of comparable incomes, *practice shift* has occurred in most states, where physicians uncertified in cosmetic procedures perform surgery to increase their incomes. Doing such surgeries outside a hospital is a loophole because more than half of states do not regulate cosmetic procedures outside hospitals.[30] Ideally, physicians who shift into other specialties should be held to the same standards of care as normal physicians in those specialties, which North Carolina recently has required.

Ultimately, the question of public policy comes down to whether physicians and customers should be *banned* from helping men and women reshape their bodies? Should society forbid people from paying physicians for aesthetic surgery, the way it forbids people from buying heroin or methamphetamine? Even Professor Little doesn't go that far, and instead urges both patients and physicians to "fight against" the tyranny of the norm.

While it may be *foolish* to pursue such values, it's hard to argue that it's *immoral*. Yes, we criticize parents who spend every evening watching their kids play sports (they have no other interests?), but it's not *immoral* to live that way. Some middle-aged singles live in St. Bart's, sailing and drinking, soaking up the sun, and just hanging out. It may be a suspect norm to live like this and not much of a life project, but that isn't immoral.

Moreover, most female clients of cosmetic surgeons do not view themselves as robots. They do not see themselves as being led by the nose of oppressive norms, but claim they deliberately chose a plan for social and professional advancement.

In addition to bodily enhancement for social and professional purposes, many people use medicine to restore their bodies after loss of function. They need such surgery after accidents from jobs, farms, and automobiles, and after falls and gunshot wounds. In addition, many people want to enhance their bodies not out of narcissism or in competition, but simply to be able to maintain their ability to work, to live independently, or to do favorite activities such as running, skiing, or bowling (hip replacements).

So suppose a woman reads all the above risks of cosmetic surgery and still wants to go ahead with, say, liposuction. Is she a fool to do so? Wasting public monies?

I believe that the range of human desires is so vast, so complex, and so individualized, that as a matter of law and morality, almost all personal enhancements should be allowed among competent adults.

So isn't Jennifer *cheating* nature, creating a false impression of herself to potential suitors, and making other women feel inferior? I think the question assumes that no one knows what Jennifer has done, whereas in most cases, it's obvious, especially when the person repeatedly pursues enhancements. The question also assumes that Jennifer isn't open about what she's done, and according to cosmetic surgeons, some women like Jennifer are not secretive about their enhancements.

Even if it wasn't obvious and Jennifer kept it secret, I don't see any great harm to others from what she's done. It's like parents hiring a private tutor so Johnny can do better on his SATs or become a better goalie in soccer. Yes, people do these things do get an advantage over others in competitions, but only the most dictatorial, intrusive state or puritanical ethics would get government involved in banning such private actions.

I agree with John Stuart Mill when he concluded in *On Liberty* that when the state forbids personal endeavors in such areas, it is very likely to do so for the wrong reasons at the wrong time and for the wrong motives. And even if justified in banning a particular case, the general principle is more important, which is that competent people should be left free to do what they want in their own lives, and modifying their bodies is about as personal as "their own lives" can get.

Nevertheless, something deeply troubles me about the secretiveness of the business of physical enhancement. I sense that thousands of women have undergone cosmetic surgery of one form or the other and that many may be unhappy. Nor do I believe that public monies should subsidize such enhancements, as in Europe, either by government programs such as Medicaid and Medicare or by group insurance.

It is difficult to find objective evidence of how happy or unhappy are the clients of cosmetic surgeons. It is not in the interest of the doctors cutting or prescribing to fund objective follow-up studies, so how do we know whether a huge percentage aren't secretly sorry they did what they did? Perhaps patients are embarrassed to admit that they tried to become more beautiful and now suffer in private or admit that they did not anticipate the number of repeated visits to the doctor's office needed to maintain their look.

If we had a national center to monitor such private enhancements, we could fund follow-up studies. We could require that a national registry be created so such studies could be done, the way we do to follow-up studies on premature babies.

Even without such a federal center, other entities could do the same. Why don't we? Consumers Union sends me a survey every year to survey how I like what I bought in cars, washing machines, and phone coverage, so why can't it survey elective surgery? Someone should be doing so.

I conclude that right now, we think about cosmetic surgery on females in an epistemic black hole. Recognizing that such enhancements are a huge business, and not knowing the long-term risks, we cannot easily evaluate them. This is an even greater problem with stealth enhancements in competitive athletics such as cycling and football, as we shall see next.

NOTES

1. John Mao, "Foot Binding: Beauty And Torture," *The Internet Journal of Biological* (2008) 1, no. 2.

2. Umberto Ecco, *History of Beauty* (New York Rizzoli, 2007).

3. Richard Reg, *Journal of Burn Care & Rehabilitation*. 23, no. 3, May/June 2002, 220.

4. Margaret Olivia Little and Susan Bordo, Erik Parens, *Enhancing Human Traits: Ethical and Social Implications (Hastings enter Studies in Ethics)* (Washington, D.C.: Georgetown University Press, 1998).

5. Frank Miller, Howard Brody & Kevin Chung, "Cosmetic Surgery and the Internal Morality of Medicine," *Cambridge Quarterly of Healthcare Ethics* 9, no. 03 (2000), 353–64.

6. Sam Dollnick, "Ethnic Differences in Plastic Surgery," *New York Times*, February 18, 2011, D13.

7. T. T. Tindholdt et al, "40 Years of Silicone Breast Implants," *Tidsskr Nor Laegeforen*, 2005 March 17; 125 (6): 79–41; M. Lehnhardt et al, "Major and Lethal Complications of Liposuction: A Review of 72 cases in Germany between 1998 and 2003," *Plastic Reconstruction Surgery* 121, no 6, June 2008, 396e–403e.

8. B. M. Coldiron et al, "Office Surgery Incidents: What Seven Years of Florida Data Show," *Dermatological Surgery* (March, 2008) 34, no.3, 285–91.

9. "The Most Popular Cosmetic Procedures," *WebMD*
http://women.webmd.com/features/most-popular-cosmetic-procedures

10. P. Trevidic, "National Survey of Deep Vein Thrombosis in Plastic and Aesthetic Surgery, Consequences and Guidelines," *Annals Chir Plastic Esthetique,* 51, no. 2, April 21, 2006, 163–69.

11. http://www.bariatric-surgery.info/statistics.htm

12. M. Lehnhardt et al, "Major and Lethal Complications of Liposuction: A Review of 72 cases in Germany between 1998 and 2003," *Plastic Reconstruction Surgery* 121, no. 6, (June, 2008), 396e–403e.

13. L. S. Toledo and R. Mauad, "Complications of Body Sculpture" Prevention and Treatment," *Clinical Plastic Surgery*, 33, no. 1, January 2006, 1–11.

14. Tom Moylan, "More than $212 Million Awarded in Botox Brain Injury Case," LexisNexis, April 29, 2011. http://www.lexisnexis.com/community/litigationresource-center/blogs/litigationblog/archive/2011/04/29/more-than-212-million-awarded-in-bo-tox-brain-injury-case.aspx

15. ClinicalTrials.gov, "Refractory Urge Incontinence and Botox Injections," http://clinicaltrials.gov/ct2/show/NCT00373789?cond=%22Urinary+Incontinence%22&rank=4

16. Robert Kolker, "The Plastic Surgeon Who Says Lip Is Basically Useless," *New York*, January 16-23, 2012, 28.

17. J. Niamtu, "Expanding Hematomas in Face-Lift Surgery: Literature Review, Case Presentations, and Caveats," *Dermatological Surgery*, 31: 9 Pt 1: September 2005, 1134-44.

18. V. Lambros and J.M. Stuzin, "The Cross-cheek Depression: Surgical Cause and Effect in the Development of the "Joker Line" and Its Treatment," *Plastic Reconstructive Surgery* 122, November 2008, 1543–52.

19. Jonathan Van Meter, "About-Face," *New York Magazine*, August 8, 2008.

20. Robert J. Fenstershelb, "Breast Implant Lawsuits," http://www.breastimplantlawsuits.com/

21. Institute of Medicine, *Safety of Silicone Breast Implants*, 1999 (Washington, D.C.; Institute of Medicine Press).

22. David Jolly and Main de la Baume, "France Recommends Removal of Suspect Breast Implants," *New York Times*, December 24, 2011, A6.

23. "France to Pay for Implants," *Birmingham News*, December 24, 2011, A3.

24. Harris (Poll) Interactive, "Patients Agree They Should Have Done More Homework Before Surgery, ASPS Survey Reveals," March 5, 2007.

25. W. Peters, "An Outcome Analysis of 100 Women after Explantation of Silicone Breast Implants," *Annals of Plastic Surgery*, 1997, July; 39, no. 1, 9–19.

26. J. K. McLaughlin, "The Safety of Silicone-Gel Breast Implants: A Review of the Epidemiological Evidence," *Annals of Plastic Surgery* 2007, Nov: 59, no. 5, 569–80.

27. Robert Kolker, "The Plastic Surgeon Who Says Lip Is Basically Useless," *New York*, January 16–23, 2012, 28.

28. C. M. McCarthy et al, "Predicting Complications following Expander/implant Breast Reconstruction: An Outcomes Analysis Based on Preoperative Clinical trials," *Plastic Reconstructive Surgery* 121, no. 6, June 2008, 1886–92.

29. J. B. Tebbets, "Achieving a Zero Percent Reoperation Rate at 3 years in a 50-consecutive-case Augmentation Mammaplasty Premarket Approval Study," *Plastic Reconstructive Surgery*, 118, no. 6, November 2006, 1453–57.

30. Jayne O'Donnell, "States Take Aim at 'Practice Drift'," *USA Today*, December 28, 2011, B1–2.

Chapter Five

Building Better Male Bodies

Male body builders often take anabolic steroids, human growth hormone, and other supplements to obtain huge masses of muscles. Consider Saul Phillips, a twenty-seven-year-old male who once considered himself frail and weak. At age seventeen, after three years of lifting weights and secretly taking anabolic steroids and human growth hormone, Saul looked like a young Arnold Schwarzenegger. He played defensive end for his high school football team, which contended for a state title. After high school, he played on a college football team that did not give out scholarships, and he continued taking steroids. After college, his use of steroids and body building continued. Many of his fellow body builders also took similar bodily enhancements.

Is there anything wrong with what Saul does? If so, what exactly is it? In our culture, some famous athletes seem to have won because they enhanced themselves. When Mark McGwire broke baseball's single-season home run record, he was taking a then-legal performance-enhancing substance. Barry Bonds took steroids for several years, probably starting in 1998, before breaking the home run record in 2001.[1]

In 1998, Tiger Woods suffered so severely from nearsightedness that, without glasses, he could barely see golf balls. Then, in October 1999, surgeons corrected his vision with lasers,[2] and he won a golf tournament. Since then, he has become famous. In 2007, he had another eye surgery.

In this chapter, I differentiate attempts to enhance human bodies into purely self-regarding cases and those involving other people. This latter kind raises moral issues because when one person enhances himself to gain a competitive edge, others are affected. For purposes of development in this chapter, I will first discuss the secret use of such substances in male-dominated sports such as football and weightlifting, and only at the end of the chapter discuss noncompetitive enhancements, such as those used by male body builders, tattoo artists, and those who suffer body-identity disorders.

One ethical issue of this chapter involves defining what consistitutes an "enhancement." Consider running a race, say, a 10,000-meter race or a half-marathon. What counts as an enhancement? Is use of a mechanical prosthesis cheating? Taking mega dosages of caffeine before the race? Using an individually-designed, tailor-made running shoe? Hiring a team to give you water and energy bars at one-mile intervals along a marathon? Using an iPod to listen to songs with a good beat (said to improve 10K times by three minutes)? A GPS device that beeps when your pace slows below your target?

In any competitive sport, coaches are enhancers.[3] Anyone with special knowledge about physiology, training, equipment, endurance, muscles, metabolism, and mental focus helps any athlete to run faster, jump higher, and win. An athlete with the wealth not to work and to hire a personal coach has enhancers. For such wealthy athletes to compete against athletes who must train after work is a kind of cheating. Ideally, everyone should start from the same place. We don't like to think of races as the chance for the wealthy to leave the poor behind, yet it sometimes is just that (swimming in the Olympic games).

A useful classification about physical enhancement and competition distinguishes between increases in performance due to technique, biology, and equipment.[4] I will not focus on technique (an example is the Fosbury flop, which transformed high-jumping in the 1960s). Instead, my discussion focuses on biological enhancements and then on equipment, such as prostheses and artificial joints.

Biological enhancements in competitive sports involve blood boosting, taking growth factors, supplements, and minerals, as well as injecting various kinds of anabolic steroids. In sports such as football, baseball, hockey, weight lifting, and body building, use of steroids is alleged to be pervasive.

The trial of Barry Bonds in 2011 publicized these issues in baseball. In 1998, Mark McGwire and Sammy Sosa battled to set the record for home runs, but something had changed. As outfielder Doug Glanville noted, he previously had a sense of how far a ball would carry and from whom, but in the early 1990s, that changed as baseballs unexpectedly sailed over fences in record numbers.[5] At the same time, Glanville said, "You were looking around and wondering how that guy got so big in the off season."

Enhancements come into play when the culture of some sports, such as professional cycling, encourages athletes to use every conceivable form of *doping* to beat the current tests. *Doping*, a term of uncertain origins, may have originated from "doop," a Dutch word Americanized as slang for a way of drugging victims, or from the South African "dop," a potent alcohol/stimulant combination. Regardless of its origins, doping has come to mean the secret use of performance-enhancing substances to gain advantage over competitors, making it synonymous with cheating.

One method of doping removes blood from an athlete's body before a competition to be stored and later returned to him before competition. Taking blood out of the body enhances the number of red blood cells because the body grows new cells to replace those lost. When the original cells are returned, the body has extra red blood cells, giving it an advantage in sports that require heavy use of oxygen, such as cycling and cross-country skiing. Training at high altitudes in the Rocky Mountains achieves the same effect because the lower concentration of oxygen stimulates the blood to create more red blood cells. Some athletes naturally possess genes that give them more red blood cells.

An athlete may also transfuse himself with the blood of others with high counts of red blood cells. Any transfer of blood runs the risk of infections, mix-ups, and contamination. If such transfusions are done to avoid detection, then the blood must be transported and given secretly and then all equipment whisked away.

So many scandals have rocked the Tour de France that it now symbolizes doping. In the 1980s, cyclists began taking the hormone erythropoietin (EPO), a hormonal growth factor that the body creates to stimulate production of red blood cells. As a medical treatment, EPO was approved for patients with anemia.

In 2006, 2007, and 2008, random testing found leading contestants with high levels of hematocrit, or the percentage of blood volume occupied by red blood cells. These high levels caused cyclists to be dismissed.[6] Several cyclists in the Tour de France later confessed to doping and claimed that every cyclist in the Tour de France also doped.

A small percentage of high school athletes—somewhere between 3 and 12 percent and a larger percentage of college and professional athletes—secretly take anabolic steroids.

Heavy usage of steroids over a decade likely harms bodies and alters personalities. The evidence has recently been building. In one study out of Harvard, the ability of the left ventricle to pump blood was compromised in users who had taken such steroids for nine years.[7] The National Institute for Drug Abuse (NIDA) states that steroid abuse damages livers, increases bad cholesterol and decreases good cholesterol, shrinks testicles, reduces sperm counts, and may lead to renal failure.[8] NIDA even claims that, in some personalities, taking anabolic steroids can be "addicting."

A special kind of steroid has been called a "designer steroid," referring to tetrahydrogestrinone (THG). Developed in a private lab called BALCO in San Francisco, THG was not available commercially and had no official uses. But the lab marketed the drug privately to star athletes such as baseball player Barry Bonds and sprinter Marion Jones. Thus it was not on the radar screens of committees testing for illegal drugs. Revelation of THG came when Jones' coach mailed THG to authorities.[9]

Some athletes believe that the dangers of using steroids are exaggerated and, in particular, that if steroids are used correctly and in moderation, they pose few risks to health. Such athletes believe that ideology biases the public's view. They liken it to medical marijuana, where people may be pro or con before they learn the facts.

Nevertheless, the practice of taking several steroids together, known as *stacking*, carries special dangers. Physicians have reported several cases where young male body builders took massive amounts of steroids and damaged their livers or hearts, or became violent. In America, so-called professional wrestling, which is really body building and acting, has witnessed several cases of "roid rage," as when professional wrestler Chris Benoit in 2007 strangled his wife, suffocated his seven-year-old son, and hanged himself with a weight-machine pulley.[10]

The secrecy of such usage makes it difficult to evaluate. Without oversight by a reputable physician or careful monitoring, it is impossible to know how many athletes take steroids. Unfortunately, because an athlete suspects that his or her competitors use steroids, it motivates him not only to take them, but also to take them in increasingly large dosages. The attitude of "I would rather win a Super Bowl ring and be dead at forty than be a loser" also motivates taking extraordinary dosages.

In one of the more bizarre stories about steroids, a reporter in New Jersey revealed that 248 police officers and firefighters were illegally supplied anabolic steroids by a forty-five-year-old physician, Joseph Colao, who appeared to have transformed himself by taking such steroids and who suddenly died in 2010 of heart failure.[11] "The use of performance-enhancers among first responders has been a taboo topic since it first came to light during the 1980s," said University of Texas professor John Hoberman in response to the article, who called the problem a national one that "has been systematically ignored" for two decades.

Although what people do to their own bodies outside competitive sports is largely their own concern, especially in taking medical risks to look muscular, a troubling aspect of this story is that Dr. Colao colluded with these men to get group medical coverage to pay for the steroids. Although less than 1 percent of men suffer from any hormonal condition requiring steroids, Dr. Colao certified all these men as such. This bilks public monies in support of unsafe, dubious norms.

Lyle Azado's story haunts discussions of professional athletes taking steroids. He played fifteen seasons as defensive end for the Denver Broncos, Cleveland Browns, and Los Angeles Raiders.[12] In college in 1969, to be a bigger football player, he began experimenting with anabolic steroids and never stopped. After receiving radical chemotherapy and contracting pneumonia, Alzado died at age forty-three in 1992. Officially, he died from brain lymphoma, a rare form of cancer.

Although steroids cannot be proven to cause brain lymphoma, Alzado himself believed that the drugs had caused his cancer. At the height of his use of enhancing drugs, Alzado estimated that he spent $30,000 a year on steroids and human growth hormone, often buying them at gyms around the country. His second wife, Cindy, blamed the breakup of their marriage on mood swings that steroids caused, a pattern also seen in wrestler Chris Benoit.

Alzado admitted the steroids made him so crazy that at times he couldn't deal with social stress. After years of denying that he used steroids and three months after being diagnosed with brain cancer, Alzado confessed in a first-person story for *Sports Illustrated* in July 1991. "It was addicting, mentally addicting," Alzado wrote on his steroid use. "I just didn't feel strong unless I was taking something." He stated that "It wasn't worth it. If you're on steroids or human growth hormone, stop. I should have."

A woman philosopher whom I once knew engaged in body building in her twenties and developed huge upper-body muscles, well outside the norms of her gender or of most men. Suspected of having taken large amounts of steroids, she died of liver failure before she reached age thirty.

If everyone was able to use steroids, there would be no benefit to taking them. Under the current situation, where only a small percentage of most athletes take steroids, a shot-putter who injects steroids can gain more muscle mass than others and thus gain a *positional advantage*. A positional advantage confers on the beneficiary an asset in a contest relative to others, but vanishes if everyone else has the same asset. If all football linemen used steroids, none would have a positional advantage. But if only one lineman uses them, he may benefit substantially.

Positional advantage matters greatly in competitive sports. Even gaining a slight advantage over opponents can make the difference between a good performance and an average one. Even when one is competing against oneself, say, in running marathons, runners go to great lengths to gain small improvements.

Citing the myriad problems of the Tour de France, Oxford University bioethicist Julian Savulescu believes that instead of trying to prohibit use of banned substances in sports, we should embrace the inevitable and legalize performance-enhancing drugs to level the playing field. For him, the enormous rewards of winning, coupled with the minimal consequences of cheating and the low chance of being caught, make doping irresistible to athletes.

Professor Savulescu thinks that drug use in elite sport is only wrong because it violates the rules, so we should change the rules. He argues that doing so will not lead to an arms race of drug-taking: "We should not think that allowing cyclists to take EPO would turn the Tour de France into some kind of 'drug race,' any more than the various training methods available turn it into a 'training race' or a 'money race.'"[13]

Savulescu thinks the only limit of drugs in sport should be safety. His opponents think the safety of athletes is a good reason for prohibiting enhancing drugs in sports, but Savulescu counters that sports like professional boxing are also unsafe and dangerous. Furthermore, banning a substance may carry its own harms. Just as prohibition of alcohol in the 1920s increased deaths due to the unregulated quality of bootleg alcohol, banning drugs in sports leads to the same problems. For Savulescu, performance enhancement retains the spirit of the sport rather than violating it.

I appreciate Professor Savulescu's arguments, but for me, the fact that we allow racecar driving and boxing does not mean that we should allow other sportive forms of bodily risk. This is the logical fallacy of *tu quo que*. Besides, perhaps we made a mistake allowing the original dangerous sports, just as we made mistakes in the twentieth century allowing everyone to smoke cigarettes.

Second, although it's *possible* that low dosages of steroids by older adults aren't harmful, most athletes take steroids and growth hormones for positional advantage not in such low dosages but in very large dosages, and finally, such usage isn't monitored by physicians. A fortiori, this is true of stacking.

Moreover, Savulescu almost admits that athletes who desire to do so will always find new drugs and new ways to take enhancers without detection. A major flaw of drug testing in Major League Baseball is that players aren't tested in the off season, when they are lifting weights and trying to gain muscle mass, and hence, most likely to take banned drugs.[14] Doctors may also give players new drugs "off label," where there is less monitoring and no testing. If so, that doesn't justify giving up on bans on steroids and other dangerous substances.

Why not? The answer is simple: because it's *cheating* to use such substances, and the question whether it's cheating fundamentally differs from whether we can catch all cheaters, whether cheaters will find innovative ways to cheat, or whether it's unsafe to cheat.

Perhaps most cyclists in the Tour de France break the rules and cheat. Does that make it ethical? Even if only a small fraction of cyclists do not cheat, an honorable way to race still exists. The appeal of American cyclist Lance Armstrong for years was partially that he did not cheat, that he beat cancer and still won, that he "lived strong" without doping.

In a tv interview on "60 Minutes" in May 2011, Lance's teammate Tyler Hamilton said he and Lance doped in the Tour de France in 1999, that Armstrong encouraged it, that he personally saw Armstrong inject himself with EPO. Hamilton said that physicians methodically gave each cyclist EPO and human growth hormone in white lunch bags, and that cyclists were driven from airports to clandestine hotel rooms where blood was taken from them to be returned to them during a race.[15]

If the majority of athletes do not cheat, then the sport maintains a dominant ethos that is still good. But when most athletes in a sport cheat—as appears to be so in the Tour de France—the entire sport becomes corrupt.

To me, the history of the Tour de France does not explain why we should legalize enhancements, but explains what happens when a culture of cheating destroys a sport. That the Tour de France has become synonymous with doping, that everyone assumes a winner to be a cheater, that sponsors decline now to endorse athletes because of tarnished images, has killed honorable, professional cycling.

Regardless of whether the practice maims your own body or kills you, taking steroids to compete is cheating, plain and simple, and the secrecy of the usage encourages stacking, as well as using greater and greater quantities, all of which justify banning use of steroids in athletic competitions. Anything not legally open to all competitors should be banned. So the controversy among users and non-users about the long-term safety of using steroids is moot. Steroids are used to gain an unfair advantage.

Of even greater importance, the casual acceptance of cheating through doping, not the use of enhancements in itself, undermines the spirit of sports and fair competition. The attitude of blatantly cheating to win has destroyed some sports. Certainly when we see a large-muscled man in body building, football, or other contact sports, we assume he's taken steroids or growth hormone. Over the last decade, the average weight of NFL linemen has increased about eighty pounds, and a lot of it is muscle. Only steroids could do that.

This same casual acceptance inside body building, cycling, and weightlifting of taking anabolic steroids and other enhancers is not a good thing. A different ethos could have evolved.

Nor is it inevitable that cheaters never get caught and that athletes will inexorably stack more and more drugs. When East German female swimmers started to look like American football players, everyone knew what was going on and it eventually stopped.

Trite as it may sound in sports, but certainly not in ethics, winning isn't everything. It's how you win, and taking banned drugs isn't the way we want our children and friends to win.

Consider also that if we allowed steroids, doping, and other supplements, as Savulescu argues, there is little evidence that, given the pervasive culture of cheating, athletes would suddenly stop cheating. If the *whole culture* is secretly injecting enhancement drugs to gain endurance and positional advantage, then that secret culture is not going to go away overnight. Legal drugs will become the baseline and new drugs will be sought for positional advantage.

Moreover, an Exposure Effect occurs in legalizing banned drugs in sports. Yes, 10 percent of football players in the United States use steroids, but if steroids were allowed, 90 percent would. And with that greater public exposure, and probably stacking, many more problems would occur.

We shouldn't harangue high school athletes about the dangers of using steroids. They will hear the opposite from older, successful athletes in college or elsewhere. Rather, we should also emphasize that it's cheating and that to use steroids is to undermine the essence of the sport.

I believe that the link between enhancement and cheating is the master philosophical question of all enhancement ethics. The idea that enhancement is cheating underlies the idea that enhancement is, if not immoral, then indicative of erroneous personal values.

Let's consider a related issue about cheating and enhancement in sports, namely the role of the physician who supplies banned drugs. If athletes taking enhancers are cheating, then physicians who provide enhancers to athletes are corrupt. Although medicine is too elastic to rigidly uphold any distinction between therapy and research—where one is a proper, the other, an improper, goal of medicine, it is not too elastic to ignore the distinction between what is in the rules and what is not. Arne Lundqvist writes that providing banned prescription drugs to healthy adults is "medical malpractice." That is too strong for most drugs, e.g., Viagra, but not for purposes of breaking the rules in competitive sports to gain positional advantage.

Another important issue in the general area of the ethics of bodily enhancement concerns use of external equipment. All equipment can be enhancing, and the best equipment offers the best enhancement. In the same way, the best running shoes and clothes require money and help the best runners. So, if you're serious about running, eventually you find a way to buy such shoes and equipment.

Of course, some nations possess good athletes in some sports only because citizens can afford Olympic-size swimming pools or have access to the money, time, and mountains to learn how to ski. This is a good example of cheating by citizens of developed nations in competing in, say, the Olympics, against citizens of developing nations. What good is it to be proud of your swimmers when most people in most developing countries lack swimming pools or the leisure time to train in them? Let's give every country a dozen Olympic-size pools, subsidize a hundred athletes to train there, and *then* see who wins the Olympic swimming medals.

It's one thing to implant an artificial lens in your eye so that you can see better or a joint in your hip so that you can walk better, but what if you do so to compete better? What is allowed and what is cheating?

Consider Oscar Pistorius, the Australian who was born with deformed feet and whose parents chose carbon blades called "Cheetahs" for him. Oscar became so good at sprinting that it became a serious ethical issue for the International Olympic Committee as to whether he could compete in the 2008 summer games in Beijing or in the 2012 games in London. He had gone from being *disabled* to *too-abled*. Ultimately, like single-amputee Sarah Reinersten, he was allowed to compete to try out for the South African team. In 2012, he hoped to win the London summer Olympics and in doing so, be the highlight of that competition.

After a 1976 water-skiing accident, Van Phillips, aged fifty-four, lost his leg below the knee, leading him to develop the prosthesis used by Pistorius. Obviously a genius, his need fused with intellect to think creatively and in doing so, he started a Copernican Revolution in rehabilitative medicine.

> Phillips said he became obsessed with creating a better prosthetic leg. ... He learned that the artificial limb industry had changed little since World War II and the Korean War. Most prosthetics were designed within the cosmetic envelope — a prosthetic foot resembled the human foot. There was no energy to propel a leg. Borrowing concepts from pole-vaulting, the spring of a diving board and the C shape of a Chinese sword his father owned, Phillips imagined a prosthetic that would let him jump and land. The result was the Flex-Foot, which

included many designs of prosthetics for a range of people. One of the designs, the Cheetah, was intended for elite athletes. ... He used carbon graphite, which is stronger than steel and lighter than aluminum. [16]

Along the way, Phillips realized that previous designers of prosthetics had mistakenly tried to replicate human bones. He realized that

"you can't function unless you have a *power source*," (my emphasis), Phillips said. He studied ligaments that store muscle energy, observing the tendons of porpoises, kangaroos and cheetahs, noting how the cheetah's hind leg landed and compressed, and the elastic nature of it. ... Paddy Rossbach, president and chief executive of the Amputee Coalition of America, said: "Van Phillips's foot changed the whole field of prosthetics. It was an extraordinary change." Sarah Reinersten, now 33, said that when she switched from a hollow wooden leg to a Flex-Foot at age 12, it felt as if "I was walking on a cloud." In 2005, she became the first female amputee to complete the Ironman triathlon.

But was it fair that Oscar could compete? I don't think it was because Pistorius was using his Cheetahs to get an extra advantage unavailable to other runners. He was RoboCop entering a shooting contest for police officers. That he was formerly disabled is irrelevant. What matters is that he was now using substances (graphite) that were stronger and more flexible than human bone, and using them to run faster. More importantly, doing so gave him an artificial source of power that natural runners lack.

I do not believe that athletes enhanced this way should compete against the non-enhanced, even if they were once disabled. It's not fair that some run on materials stronger than bones and with an ability to spring the runner forward.

In 1998, Casey Martin, a twenty-five-year-old golfer with a disability wanted to ride a golf cart between holes rather than walk. A federal judge ruled that he could compete on the professional golf tour and ride his cart. Does the game of golf simply consist of driving the ball, putting, and expertly shaving par into birdies and hole-in-one shots? Of course not! Endurance, and specifically walking, factors into the sport because the more tired the golfer is, the harder it is for him to hit accurately and far. Long ago, professional golfers abandoned carrying their own bags, employing caddies instead. That was the beginning of ending golf as a real athletic event, but at least every professional golfer can have a caddy.

Some disagree with my view. Among the people rooting for Pistorius is Hugh Herr of MIT's biomechatronics lab, who said of Oscar's Olympic competition,[17] "the minute an athlete with an unusual body or mind becomes competitive, they're a threat. Before that happens, they're seen as cute or courageous. Once they win, they're accused of cheating."[18]

In both the case of Oscar Pistorius and of Casey Martin, sympathy for a person with a disability resulted in the wrong decision to allow them to compete with a superior advantage. That is, they were allowed to cheat because they had a disability. The same reasoning should allow the blind to compete in archery by using finger-initiated laser trails to guide their arrows to the target.

My central argument against the common use of enhancements in competitions is not an indirect one but a direct one: enhancements are wrong because they are cheating. Cheating in competitions is wrong. Widespread cheating corrupts the sport and renders its prizes meaningless.

What, then, about Saul Phillips, the twenty-seven-year-old, single, competent male who has transformed his body over the last decade from a stick-like Ichabod Crane to a muscle-bound Hulk? He is ripped. Where previously Saul despised his body and women scared him, he now proudly exhibits his body and seeks the company of women. Like Jennifer in the last chapter, when he sees people staring at him, he enjoys it.

Is he a cheater, too, like the cyclists on the Tour de France? In my opinion, he's only cheating like Jennifer, and if so, only in a very small sense. Like Jennifer, he may be only fooling himself if he thinks everyone else believes he achieved his muscles naturally. Like some Jennifers, he may freely admit to others that he didn't achieve his bodily results naturally. But when these men enter bodybuilding competitions, they are cheating. The way they look and their ability to lift weights or pose is only partly due to their efforts. The other part is due to the substances they take secretly and, if not all others take the same substances, then they have an unfair advantage.

Second, given the medical dangers discussed in the beginning of this chapter, physicians who enable such men to bulk up are corrupt. Fake bodily enhancement is a two-way illicit street, brining down both those who prescribe and those who get steroids, growth hormones, and other muscle-producing substances.

Consider a different kind of enhancement, one that calls into question the definition of the term. If Enthusiasts subscribe to the Anything Goes view that physicians and competent males should be able to do anything they want to their bodies, so long as it doesn't harm others, then what about tattoos? One in fourteen people in North America and Europe sports a tattoo; tattoos cover significant portions of some people's bodies. Other people may find such extensive tattoos offensive, even repulsive. Although people may not realize it, the skin is also an organ, and tattoos may inflict long-term damage on the skin's ability to protect the body from assaults.

Yet their owners usually think of tattoos as embellishments. Is one person's disfigurement another's beauty? Why else would such people spend considerable amounts of money to obtain the tattoos, sit under a needle for hours while the tattooist stains their skin, and undergo minor pain? In the same way, others sport metallic jewelry surgically implanted on various parts of their bodies. One woman's blemish is another's trophy.

Obviously, whether to permanently color one's skin in patterned ways is a personal issue and one that only minimally affects other people. Those offended can look away, just as they don't have to read every bumper sticker or every salacious book cover. Of course, it's reasonable that medical insurance and state funds don't pay for tattoos.

But how far should physicians go with bodily modifications? Consider also Cat Man, aka John Doe, who has had his face modified to look feline, including having his teeth sharpened to resemble a cat's incisors, whiskers implanted, and eyebrows changed. He thinks he looks good, but his looks repel others. *Chacun à son goût?*

No matter what we think about tattoos or Cat Man, such bodily self-modifications rest in the area of aesthetics, not morality. We may dispute whether having your body covered with tattoos counts as beautiful, but some think so. So long as no one is harmed by such tattoos, or sharpened teeth, it's just personal aesthetics.

What about amputation envy or *apotemnophilia*, officially *body integrity disorder (BID)*.[19] Portrayed on medical dramas such as *Grey's Anatomy*, *CSI: New York*, and *Nip/Tuck*, as well as in the book, *Geek Love*, subjects commonly yearn intensely to have a leg amputated above the left knee. Although almost all surgeons refuse to operate this way, at least one surgeon in Scotland has amputated legs of two competent patients.[20] Assuming such patients are competent, does such amputation really benefit them?

Within days after a suspicious amputation in Tijuana, Philip Bondy, a seventy-eight-year-old retired satellite engineer, who suffered for years from apotemnophilia, died from gangrene in 1998. The surgeon who amputated Bondy's legs was John Ronald Brown, dubbed by one documentary as "The Worst Doctor in America," for botching surgeries involving penis enlargement, sex reassignment, and apotemnophilia. But as one author states, "Bondy's case is illustrative of both the grim determination of apotemnophiles to effectuate the amputations they desire and the serious physical harm to which this determination makes them potentially vulnerable."

■■■

If this chapter leaves the reader with a sleazy feeling about males enhancing their bodies, and the physicians who enable such males, so be it. The combination of direct payment, off-label prescribing, and stealth muscle building has been dangerous for many men. It is a dangerous norm building up in sports, one that may corrupt them. The conviction of Barry Bonds in April 2011, for obstructing justice in an investigation of his taking banned steroids, shows how low the sport of professional baseball has fallen, joining the Tour de France in the Hall of Shame.

NOTES

1. Mark Fairnau-Wade and Lance Williams, *Game of Shadows: Barry Bonds, BAL-CO, and the Steroids Scandal that Rocked Professional Sports* (New York: Gotham, 1997).

2. Woods Has Second Laser Eye Surgery," *Golf Tours and News*, May 15, 2007. http://www.golf.com/golf/tours_news/article/0,28136,1621439,00.html

3. Early Olympic rules about amateurs once attempted to exclude coaches and limit amount of time practiced.

4. I owe this distinction to Julian Savulescu, Nick Bostrom (eds). *Human Enhancement* (London: Oxford University Press, 2009).

5. Kristen Merriweather, *Epoch* News Staff, December 23–28, 2011, B4 (Washington, D.C.).

6. Jamey Keaten, "Tour Rocked Again by Doping," Associated Press, July 18, 2008, *Birmingham News*, D8.

7. Aaron L. Baggish et al, "Long Term Anabolic-Androgenic Steroid Use is Associated with Left Ventricular Dysfunction," *Circulation and Heart Failure* 109, April 27, 2010.

8. NIDA Info-Facts; Steroids. http://www.drugabuse.gov/infofacts/steroids.html .

9. Julian Savulescu and Bennett Foddy, "Le Tour and the Failure of Zero Tolerance: Time to Relax Doping Controls," in *Enhancing Human Capacities*, ed. Julian Savulescu, Ruud ter Meulen & Guy Kahane (London: Wiley-Blackwell, 2011), 305.

10. Associated Press, "Cops Eye 'Roid Rage' in Wrestler's Murder-Suicide," June 27, 2007.

11. Amy Brittan and Mark Mueller, "New Jersey Doctor Supplied Steroids to Hundreds of Law Enforcement Officers, Firefighters," *New Jersey Star-Ledger*, March 9, 2010.

12. http://espn.go.com/classic/biography/s/Alzado_Lyle.html

13. Julian Savulescu et al, "Why We Should Allow Performance Enhancing Drugs in Sport," *British Journal of Sports Medicine*, 38 (2004), 666–70.

14. Daniel Pauling, "MLB Drug Testing Doesn't Cut it," letter, *Birmingham News*, May 23, 2011, D2.

15. "Who Is Tyler Hamilton?" *60 Minutes*, May 20, 2011.

16. Carol Pogash, "A Personal Call to a Prosthetic Invention," *New York Times*, July 2, 2008.

17. Herr quoted in Rowan Philip, "Oscar Could Be Fastest Man," *TIME*, January 29, 2012.

18. A. A. Lawrence. "Clinical and Theoretical Parallels between Desire for Limb Amputation and Gender Identity disorder," *Archives of Sexual Behavior, 25,* (2006), 263–78.

19. Annemarie Bridy, "Confounding Extremities: Surgery at the Medico-Ethical Limits of Self-Modification," *Journal of Law, Medicine & Ethics*, 32, 2004.

20. Annemarie Bridy, "Confounding Extremities."

Chapter Six

Is It Moral to Feel Better than Well?

"In the depths of the depression, getting a stamp on a letter is a day's work."
— Talk show host Dick Cavett, describing his life-long depression

In 1935, Borden, the maker of milk products, produced a famous animated cartoon called "the Sunshine Makers." It featured one group of grumpy dwarfs who went around saying, "I'm sad" or "I feel terrible," and another happy group that would reply, "That's good!" The happy group, filled with sunshine, tries to get the sad group to be happy by firing guns loaded with sunshine at them, but the Grumpies resist. In the end, the Happies bombard the Grumpies with sunshine, and after being forced to be happy, the Grumpies rejoice.

Alarmists think that an alliance of pharmaceutical companies and psychiatrists push sunshine on a society of passive Grumpies, and that such techie sunshine cannot substitute for the real thing. In *Beyond Therapy: Biotechnology and the Pursuit of Happiness*, Leon Kass implies that such sunshine merely mimics authentic life. Yes, you can take Prozac to feel better, but it's a drug-induced fog.

Kass' view mimics one of the greatest works of literature about mood-altering drugs, Aldous Huxley's *Brave New World*. A benevolent dictatorship runs a highly efficient society stratified by biological castes, where a daily dose of Prozac-like *soma* keeps citizens quiescent. If citizens take too much soma, it puts them to sleep.

The opposite of *Brave New World* appeared in 2007 when psychiatrist Peter Kramer published *Listening to Prozac.* In it, he describes Tess, a woman in her mid-thirties in public housing who, after her father died when she was twelve, cared for her depressed mother and her nine siblings, never dating and always living for others.[1] She came to Dr. Kramer depressed and unable to socialize. On Prozac, Tess overcame her depression and fears, started to date, left her apartment, and became independent.

Critics claim that the Prozac engendered fake happiness for Tess. Tess retorted to Kramer that Prozac allowed her real self to appear.

Kramer reports that many of his patients experienced the same thing. In a chapter entitled "Makeover," he describes how patients on Prozac lost their compulsivity or depression, became focused, and no longer avoided people.

Clinical depression, as opposed to the passing depression of temporary setbacks, has been described by some as feeling like being in a cold, dark freezer that numbs emotions. Antidepressants such as Prozac take one out of the freezer and into the sunshine.

Critics say the hard way of talking therapy is better, but why, I wonder, is the more difficult way better? Is it more effective? Traditional talking psychotherapy works well for some problems, but not for depression caused by biochemical imbalance. Because our Puritan heritage makes us think we don't deserve to be happy, do we mistrust quick fixes?

For critics of mood enhancement, antidepressants symbolize enhancement. They represent quick, shallow change. Where natural change of mood comes slowly and arduously, change with antidepressants seems quick and easy. For critics, if we become a Prozac Nation, we'll morph into drugged zombies who shuffle around blandly on islands of Dr. Moreau. On antidepressants, we'll spend our days atrophying on the Internet, prisoners in Plato's Cave, watching shadows of pixelated artifacts.

Some bioethicists, such as philosopher Carol Freedman of Williams College, philosopher Erik Parens of the Hastings Institute, and Minnesota physician Carl Elliott, argue that mood enhancers enforce dubious norms, undermine personal responsibility, and substitute a false, manufactured personality for earned character. This character only comes through effort and struggle. As such, these bioethicists favor public policy that limits such drugs.[2]

Wake Forest English professor Eric Wilson, in *Against Happiness: In Praise of Melancholy,* leads this charge from the brigade of literature. He argues that Prozac simulates a living death, blocks our creativity, hinders our spiritual-growth-through-suffering, and should be avoided.[3] Wilson believes that creativity, success, ambition, and vision conflict with a desire to be happy, and that this desire for happiness will lead us into "half-lives, to bland existences, to wastelands of mechanistic behavior."[4] For Wilson, to be happy at all, while people die in Africa from AIDS, is to be "inauthentic." Sorrow is "sweet," he says, but happiness is "self-satisfied smiles" (smugness), "treacly expressions ... painted on our faces" like botoxed lips and rouge. To be happy is to have "an essential part of [our] hearts sliced away and discarded like so much waste."

So should we go forth and suffer? Should we wish on Wilson, then, an unhappy, turbulent, chaotic life? According to Wilson's writings, we should. Here Wilson taps into an ancient Christian trope of growth-through-suffering, itself an answer to the age-old Problem of Evil (Question: Why do we suffer so much from a kindly God? Answer: He wants us to grow in spirit.)

Perhaps the best, shortest attack on Wilson's book comes from comedian-singer Garrison Keillor, producer of National Public Radio's "Prairie Home Companion." In a review of Wilson's book, Keillor wondered why, given that Wilson embraced suffering so much, he hadn't written a better book.[5]

When it comes to mild depression, anxiety, and other mood disorders, philosopher Freedman argues that it's a *fact* that talking therapy beats drugs.[6] However, a review of the clinical literature does not appear to back up her claim.[7]

Carl Elliott agrees with Wilson and argues that mild depression should not be seen as an illness but as a personal reaction to the ills of the world. "From this perspective," he says, "treatment of the depressing state should not be covered by insurance because the condition is actually a truth about the world."[8]

Elliott is clear about what values may be lost using Prozac. He thinks people should ideally have a long-term project in life toward which they work and the completion of which fulfills them. Part of this quest comes from looking inward and searching for a worthy project. Elliott considers a suburban accountant who, while seeing a psychiatrist, questions his life. Elliott thinks that if the accountant gets Prozac, he will stop questioning his life because he has been contentedly medicated, so the psychiatrist should not write him a prescription.

I agree with Elliott about the ideal. Unfortunately, most people find it difficult to obtain. Even with effort, good health, secure income, and intelligence, it takes luck.

The assumption that Alarmists make is that projects performed on mood enhancers *are fake*. They think that the good results come from a drug, not one's true self.

I personally believe that for many people, a biochemical disturbance lies behind their depression. So I believe that any increase in happiness they achieve on antidepressants is real, not fake.

Remember Dick Cavett and his talk show, where he sparkled with the world's wittiest guests. Many were shocked to read in 2008 that Cavett suffers from severe depression. In his essay in the *New York Times*, Cavett urges people not to ask the sufferer "what he has to be depressed about," because the illness is biochemical, not situational. [9]

Cavett wished that his psychiatrist could once get inside him for a minute to feel what he felt. When his psychiatrist heard this, he replied, "Oh, I know. I got pretty sad when my father died." To which Cavett angrily retorted, "Do you think grief is even close to this?" He went on to describe how bad things can get:

> … when you're downed by this affliction, if there were a curative magic wand on the table eight feet away, it would be too much trouble to go over and pick it up. There's also the conviction that it may have worked for others but it wouldn't work for you. Your brain is busted and nothing's going to help. … In the depths of the depression, getting a stamp on a letter is a day's work.

So would English professor Wilson urge Cavett to stay creative and eschew anti-depression drugs?

No, he and the other bioethicists say we can allow such drugs for people with severe depression. Critics fight not over genuine clinical depression but over mild depression, the kind that may be temporary, a life-stage (post-partum depression), or situational (after being fired), and which millions struggle with during part of their lives. For such mild depression, Wilson thinks people should avoid antidepressants.

Of course it makes sense that Wilson is an English professor. English, especially because of its subfield of creative writing, has become a popular, ersatz therapy for people with mental illness. Some mistaken person often encourages these vulnerable people to write about their delusions as therapy. In fact, this is only true if the writer adopts a third-person perspective, if he does not relive violent episodes, and if the professor of creative writing has been trained in supervising the writing of people with mental illnesses, all rarely the case. [10]

After the Virginia Tech shootings in 2007, English professors across North America worried about whether students who showed potential for violence should be expelled from class. The shooter, Seung-Hui Cho, wrote about violent acts in poet Nikki Giovanni's class.

In January 2008, the Association of Writers and Writing Programs at their annual meeting in New York City held a special session devoted to this topic. The session concluded that Wilson's view does not help many troubled people: these people need good drugs, psychiatrists, and reality checks, not encouragement to throw away their medications.

The strangest thing about this debate is the notion of other people judging one person's private mental states. What could it possibly be more difficult? Or more obnoxious than some know-it-all telling Martha that, although Martha has never felt more at the top of her game as a history professor, Martha teaches inauthentically because she takes antidepressants?

Here's why Wilson is wrong. If antidepressants made thirty million Americans into zombies, wouldn't it be obvious to the rest of us that their lives had turned into *Night of the Living Dead?* On the other hand, if we have the repeated testimony of many who take antidepressants that their lives improved greatly, that they couldn't imagine going back to life without drugs, and that they now *function* better as mothers, editors, and teachers, then these observations do not sound like those of zombies but of awakened Rip Van Winkles.

Perhaps Wilson confuses old and new drugs. Old-time antidepressants made people zombie-like, but new ones let personality spring forth. As Emory bioethicist Paul Wolpe observes, in both cases the new person may be unrecognizable to those who once knew her. [11]

A critic might ask me why I favor allowing people to somatize their moods with Prozac while I question Virtual Life and cosmetic surgery as fake. Well, I believe that major clinical depression is a biochemical disorder like schizophrenia and, as such, should be treated biochemically. That is, I don't believe that most depression is fake or that its cure is fake.

I view the history of psychiatry as a fight against the view that merely better attitudes can cure mental illness. Whether it is better attitudes by parents to avoid an Oedipal complex in boys, or better attitudes of depressed patients to will themselves to "snap out of it," society has often believed that something softer than biology causes mental illness.

When biology faces free will as the cause of diseases, biology usually wins. We once thought that only the sinful got syphilis, cholera, and HIV, but now we know better. We once thought that people's attitudes caused depression, bipolar disease, sexual orientation, and schizophrenia, but now we know better.

Popular wisdom has made many mistakes about mental illness and will likely continue to do so. Public policy about reimbursement of treatment for mental illness has fared even worse: few systems of medical coverage adequately cover such problems. This error began decades ago when some critics thought people with schizophrenia, in order to get out of work and to get benefits, faked their delusions.

Such mistakes show that we are as likely to be wrong as correct in thinking that competent adults fare better off antidepressants than on them. Given that chance of error, why shouldn't group policies cover them?

A mean, cold-hearted worldview mistakenly substitutes a personal view of goods in one worldview with a just public policy. The personal worldview is that antidepressants for mild depression are frivolous, unworthy of being subsidized by group medical coverage.

Only a few decades ago, everyone thought that psychiatrists could use therapy to talk people out of being depressed. Of course, legions of counselors, social workers, therapists, and clergy still make a living through talk therapy. They believe it's the only way.

But as Peter Kramer said about Tess, that view just begs the question. If competent judges—who've experienced both states—claim the drugs helped them, then critics are mistaken.

Critics such as Wilson do not empathize with the situational depression of a single mother who works the night shift of KFC at an interstate gas station, feeling trapped, and going nowhere. Maybe she needs antidepressants to keep putting food on the table. Until the revolution comes and its workers' paradise, maybe she could use some "inauthentic" happiness? Would it be so terrible for her physician to help her? Or should she take Wilson's advice and, for the good of her soul, suffer?

The reality is that she will be lucky to have any medical coverage, much less for mental illness, much less for antidepressants. Employers out to maximize profit don't offer employees coverage for mental illness or coverage for the drugs such people need to function.

Many people's lives fare less-than-ideal, as they try to cope with deaths of pets, children, spouses, and aging parents, and also endure job stress, personal illness, and poverty. Some were laid off or never found good, profitable careers. Still others remain in bad relationships for the sake of children or finances.

In the end, does it matter whether a lousy life changed Gene's biochemistry or whether Gene's lousy biochemistry caused Gene's unhappy life? In either case, improving the biochemistry may change the way Gene *feels* about this life.

I am rarely depressed and I don't take anti-depressants, but perhaps my biochemistry will change in ten years and I will need them. I certainly might need them if situational trauma, such as the death of someone I love, changed my biochemistry.

In conclusion, our method of analyzing different kinds of cases has paid off in this chapter. We shouldn't lump all enhancement-physicians together. Psychiatrists prescribing antidepressants to depressed people differ ethically from sleazy physicians prescribing growth hormone to every client who enters their office with a roll of $100 bills. Ideally, it's best not to need any enhancement, but life is not always ideal, and for many people—and perhaps each of us one day—it's nice to have such tools around when we need them.

NOTES

1. Peter D. Kramer, *Listening to Prozac* (New York: Viking, 1993), 1ff.
2. Ronald Bailey, *Liberation Biology: The Scientific and Moral Case for the Biotech Revolution* (Amherst, NY: Prometheus, 2005), 234.
3. Eric Wilson, *Against Happiness: In Praise of Melancholy* (New York: Farrar, Straus and Giroux, 2009).
4. Eric Wilson, *Against Happiness*, 6.
5. Garrison Keillor, "'Against Happiness': What Goes Up Should Come Down," review of *Against Happiness*, *International Herald Tribune*, March 14, 2008. http://www.iht.com/articles/2008/03/11/arts/IDSIDE15.php
6. Carol Freedman, in Erik Parens (ed), *Enhancing Human Traits: Ethical and Social Implications*, (Washington, D.C.: Georgetown University Press, 1998).
7. See the National Institutes for Mental Health web page on "Depression" and notes 21–27: http://www.nimh.nih.gov/health/publications/depression/complete-index.shtml

8. James Sabin, review of *Enhancing Humans*, ed. Erik Parens, *Journal of Health Politics, Policy and Law*, 26:4, August 2001, 809.

9. Dick Cavett, "Smiling Through," *New York Times*, June 27, 2008.

10. "Teaching the Troubled: Writing Workshops after Virginia Tech," Association of Writers and Writing Programs (meeting), New York City, February 2, 2008.

11. Quoted by Ronald Bailey in *Liberation* Biology, 234.

Chapter Seven

Ways to Build a Longer Life

This chapter focuses on increasing longevity and efforts to cure age-related diseases. The following chapter discusses how these advances may affect us socially.

For centuries, futurists predicted that science would offer humans longer lives; Enthusiasts predicted that science would conquer death. Within the past two generations, medicine has put some meat on those predictive bones, extending lives of citizens by twenty years in developed countries .

The longest documented human life belonged to Jeanne Calment, a Frenchwoman who died in 1997 at 122. Next came a Japanese woman, Shigechiyo Izumi, who lived to 120, followed by Americans Sarah Knauss, 119, Canadian Marie-Louise Meilleur, 118, and Lucy Hannah, 117.[1] The Gerontology Research Group of the *Guinness Book of Records* verified that over one hundred humans, all women, have lived to 113.[2]

Researchers at Mt. Sinai Hospital in New York study dozens of SuperAgers in New York City, a cohort of Ashkenazic Jews who commonly live well beyond 100 years. They seem to possess four genes that protect against cancer, cardiovascular disease and diabetes, dementia, and atherosclerosis.[3] The expected results, combined with a blood test for the length of telomeres at mid-age, may create a blood test that predicts when your body will fall apart.[4]

In 2006, 2.4 million Americans died; 4.7 million newborns replaced them.[5] According to the U.S. Census Bureau, by June 2008, the world had 6.7 billion humans.[6] Every year, 80 million more people begin life on Earth than leave it (135 million begin, 55 million leave). As such, world population by 2012 should reach 7 billion.

For the average human, expected longevity improved from an estimated twenty-five years in 15,000 B.C. to thirty-five years in the time of Sparta. In the United States, expected longevity has improved from forty-seven years in 1900 to sixty-five years in 1950 to seventy-five years in 1990 to eighty years in 2011.[7]

Over the past 160 years, American longevity has increased about 2.5 years per decade. Women generally outlive men by three years. For future women, expected longevity at age 50 will be 88 years in 2024 and 100 years in 2104.[8] (More later on these amazing facts and what they imply.)

What enables people to live longer now stems from progress started long ago. To strengthen his country, Otto von Bismarck, Prime Minister of Prussia for the latter half of the nineteenth century, started many reforms in public health, such as mandatory public sanitation, clean water, and public education. Physician Rudolf Virchow had already taught the view that better social and economic conditions could improve the health of citizens, a view known sometimes as "social medicine." Together, Virchow and Bismarck revolutionized thinking about health and longevity. In 1883, Bismarck also founded a national pension system for old age and decided that retirement began at age sixty-five, an age still used—perhaps incorrectly—in America today for eligibility for Medicare.

Bismarck's and Virchow's ideas, along with other advances, helped increase longevity, especially clean water and sanitation, vaccinations, acceptance of the germ theory of disease around 1900, discovery of antibiotics in the 1940s, improved occupational safety, and defeat of lethal childhood illnesses. Simple things such as seat belts, lower speed limits, and cars with multiple air bags also helped.

Human longevity increased in developed countries by stacking lots of big and small improvements. I shall return to this fact at the end of this chapter, but first I want to consider prospects for rapid increases in longevity or even a cure for death.

■■■

Biologist Leonard Hayflick discovered in 1965 that the maximal human life span is fixed at about 125 years. Doubling that would be a feat requiring stupendous discoveries and a fantastic commitment by the public to fund new research in biology.

Why is it so difficult to cure aging at the cellular level? A basic fact of biology is that cells can only divide so many times (about fifty). Cells have a built-in destiny to die at some point, an event called *apoptosis*. Telomeres, like the plastic caps on the ends of shoelaces, keep our cellular shoelaces from fraying. Each time a cell replicates through mitosis, its telomeres shorten.

How many times telomeres can shorten before they die (enter senescence) is their *Hayflick limit*, named for Hayflick's discovery of this fact.[9] Cells of different species have different Hayflick limits and, hence, different life spans.

The enzyme telomerase keeps telomeres healthy and appears to be the key to slowing down aging at the cellular level. Why not give cells more telomerase, restoring what telomeres lose in mitosis, and stop cellular aging?

Unfortunately, doing so would probably cause cancer. Forcing a cell to die (when its telomeres are too short) keeps it from growing out of control (cancer is essentially this). When cells replicate, DNA on the tips can mutate and become unstable. While this happens all the time, the p53 gene kills out-of-control cells, stopping cancer in the body by shortening the cell's telomeres and making the cancerous cell die.[10] Thus, if you prevent telomeres from shortening and block the p53 gene's action, you prevent the body from stopping cancer. UAB biology professor Trygve Tollefsbol, an expert on aging and telomeres, says, "Aging can be seen as a tumor suppressor mechanism."[11]

Hayflick distinguished between trying to reverse aging at the cellular level and trying to cure age-related diseases. He claims that if we cured cardiovascular disease, cancer, and stroke, we would only increase life expectancy by fifteen years.[12]

Hayflick's distinction is valuable. For one thing, he criticizes the conflation of research into aging-related diseases with research to stop aging. The latter goal, obviously, is much more difficult to achieve. The distinction also allows us to make another, namely between life span and life expectancy. The human species' maximal life span may be 125 years, but the average human life expectancy is far less than that. If nothing else, modern medicine could move us closer to our optimal life span.

Conquering aging at the cellular level would be a momentous undertaking. It would require a commitment of resources like those for building the Panama Canal or putting a man on the moon. To do so would take tremendous political will and public consensus.

Nevertheless, breakthroughs could occur. In 1996, textbooks of cellular biology stated that it was a law of nature that once cells became differentiated, they could not be returned to a pluripotent state. Steed Willadsen proved that wrong, opening the doors to not only the cloning of Dolly but also knowledge of stem cells.[13] Others later discovered adult stem cells and idiopathic pluripotent stem cells—all of which were previously unknown. As this book went to press, two major studies in mice, one about a drug that reduces fat in livers and increases sensitivity to insulin (SRT-1720,), and another about a discovery of senescent cells, hoped to be seminal breakthroughs that might one day translate into retarding human aging at the cellular level.[14]

We should keep an open mind about fixed limits and continue studying.

■■■

One key approach to anti-aging research is to study chemicals produced when the body starves. Rats fed 35 to 70 percent less calories live 25 to 40 percent longer. If such chemicals could be reproduced and safely injected into cells, perhaps the body could be fooled into thinking it was starving when a person ate normally.[15]

One company identified this substance as resversatrol, a substance found in the skin of red grapes. This substance lies behind the so-called "French paradox," the fact that Frenchmen eat foods high in saturated fats but have low incidences of coronary artery disease. Their consumption of resversatrol in red wine is alleged to explain this paradox, and after a segment was aired in 1991 on "60 Minutes" about this effect, consumption of red wine in America jumped 44 percent (and wine companies lobbied to label red wine a "health food"). Unfortunately, a decade of well-funded scientific studies has failed to confirm any anti-aging benefits of taking resveratrol in concentrated forms.[16]

Another chemical approach to anti-aging research is taking mega-doses of vitamins in attempts to counteract the damage caused by free radicals inside cells. Anti-aging researcher Jay Olshansky dismisses this approach as "a way to make expensive urine."[17]

To maintain muscles and to combat fragility, others inject human growth hormone, but the benefits are no better than those of exercise. Also, the dangers of injection (infection at the site) can be huge.

More philosophically, we should emphasize that most people don't want extra decades of being feeble or senile, but rather extra decades with *compression of morbidity*. We want to play tennis right up to the last month, and then have everything break down at once, like the famous one-horse shay of Oliver Wendell Holmes.[18]

Gerontologists long ago redefined aging from *chronological* criteria.[19] If a woman can do all the activities of a normal forty-year-old, why should she be classified by the old standards of what sixty-year-olds can do? Indeed, a *functional definition of aging* much more accurately represents the reality of a person's life and corresponds with what one sees in a hospital.[20] Defined by the ability to do or not to do a dozen "Activities of Daily Living" (ADLs), such as walking, driving, cleaning, and eating, these criteria much more accurately measure how old a person is. They measure how well a man can live by himself and act as humans normally do. For example, a fifty-year-old man with congestive heart failure who cannot walk to the corner is the functional equivalent of a ninety-year-old man.

But do we need drugs and surgery to live longer? A lot of medical evidence indicates that living healthfully over decades is the best way to make a body live longer. In the twenty-first century, epidemiologists can give better advice about how to do this. Consider a summary by two leading Harvard researchers of new evidence about the role of diet and exercise in preventing—not type 2 diabetes or heart disease—but cancer.[21] They write:

> We've known for a long time that a high-fat diet, obesity, and lack of exercise can increase the risk of developing heart disease and type-2 diabetes, two conditions that affect millions of Americans. What we are finding out now is that those same lifestyle factors also play an important role in cancer. That's bad news. The good news is that you can do something about your lifestyle. If we grew thinner, exercised regularly, avoided diets rich in red meat ... and ate diets rich in fruits and vegetables, and stopped using tobacco, we would prevent 70 percent of all cancers.

That's an amazing claim. *Seven in ten cancers could be prevented by relatively simple changes in how we live.* This new evidence contradicts the fatalistic view that most cancer stems from the genes. In fact, genes alone determine only a tiny percentage of breast, ovarian, and other cancers.

The evidence behind the claim is also impressive. People with the same genes, say, Asians, who adopt a Western lifestyle of no exercise, high-fat, red meat diets, and who put on pounds, suddenly start to develop breast, colon, and other cancers at the high rates found among North Americans living the same Western lifestyle.

Even people who had cancer can decrease their chances of recurrence by changing their ways. People with colon cancer who continued to eat badly, even after part of their colon was removed to excise their cancer, had three times more risk of cancer returning than people who changed their diet.

Both Alarmists and Enthusiasts often talk of the implications of a miraculous anti-aging pill, yet the implications of the evidence just presented are that this pill already exists: all we need to do is change how we live.

Marriage also factors into longevity. Marriage reduces the risks of early death and contributes to good health, especially for men.[22] (Epidemiologists dispute the exact causes: does ill health discourage marriage? Do healthier men get married easily? Are young men who marry early already healthier?)

Consider also exercise training in senior citizens that prevents loss of muscle. From age thirty to age fifty, people lose up to 10 percent of their muscle mass, but from ages fifty to eighty, they typically lose another 30 percent. One approach to preventing this loss, weight training, helps seniors retain such mass.

New studies show that weight training plans designed to stimulate synthesis of protein for growth of new muscle in young people are not as effective in those over sixty, who generally seem to have a blunted protein synthesis response to each exercise bout and appear more susceptible to muscle inflammation.[23] So how can seniors maintain muscle mass, or regrow lost muscle through exercise?

The answer lies in reducing exercise from three to two times a week and in modifying the eccentric exercises. Most injuries stem from lowering weights, not lifting them, so seniors should *lift* objects, not *lower* them.[24] According to University of Alabama at Birmingham professor of physiology Marcus Bamman, the benefits of this extra recovery time between exercise sessions for older adults likely stem from both enhanced muscle protein synthesis and stem cell activity, as well as reduced inflammation.

Beyond this modest method of reducing loss of muscle is the revolutionary proposal that each adult over fifty should get an *individualized exercise prescription*. Professor Bamman states,

> I would love for people to appreciate that an exercise prescription could be approached exactly like a drug prescription. There's a proper dosage and a time-course for it to wash out. [25]

Wow! What a great idea! Can you imagine a different kind of medicine where healthy patients had not only a primary care physician, but also a personal exercise prescription? I'm not talking about personal trainers but rather a person with an advanced degree in exercise physiology and nutrition. That is far different from our present system.

Finally, consider an issue close to enhancing mood. What if we could quickly lose weight with a pill? Would traditionalists want to ban it, arguing that we should only lose weight the approved way, through willpower, diet, and exercise? In 2008, reports emerged of a miraculous pill that, when given to mice, allegedly created the same physiological and metabolic good effects as if they had exercised. [26] If it carried over to humans, taking this pill would give people the beneficial effects of exercise without exercising. Francis Collins testified in 2002 before the President's Council of Bioethics that such a new pill "will help normal people be more svelte than they otherwise would be." [27]

Imagine that you could eat as much as you wanted and really not gain weight—perhaps because the drug metabolizes extra food in a different way, making it quickly pass through the gastrointestinal tract, or that it helps cap your serum cholesterol levels. Wouldn't that be a really different kind of life? For some people, it might even qualify as a Fukuyamaesque, post-human future. Would some women give up their humanity to eat as much as they pleased? Would some men do the same and gladly become satiated post-humans?

The most exciting development about longevity is that we may have quietly increased human longevity by a decade and nobody noticed. An exciting article by biodemographer James Vaupel in a March 2010 issue of *Nature* announced a "fundamental discovery about the biology of human aging, . . . one with profound implications for individuals, society, and the economy." [28] This discovery, first substantiated in

1994, is that more and more people in developed countries are reaching old age in good health. Not only is death being delayed, but people are getting an extra decade of functional living.

The implications of this finding will reverberate through future discussions of intergenerational ethics and public policy. Vaupel writes that "most children born since 2000 will celebrate their 100th birthday—in the twenty-second century. Longer life spans will alter the way individuals want to allocate time during their lives and will require radical revisions of employment, retirement, health, education, and other policies."[29]

As explained at the beginning of this chapter, this advance did not come from a sensational breakthrough in altering genes or some anti-aging elixir. Instead, it came about incrementally from stacking many different enhancements: "The progress made in lengthening life spans and postponing senescence is entirely due to medical and public health efforts, rising standards of living, better education, healthier nutrition, and more salubrious lifestyles."[30]

The cynic typically responds to news about increased longevity with quips such as, "Great! Two decades in a nursing home rather than one!" But the increase in longevity is not being accompanied by dysfunction and senescence: "The process of deterioration with age is not being slowed over time: it is being delayed." Moreover, "levels of mortality and other indices of health that used to prevail at age 70 now prevail at age 80, and levels that used to prevail at age 80 now prevail at age 90."

Other evidence seems to confirm this trend. According to a 2000 Harris poll conducted by the National Council on Aging, half of Americans ages sixty-five to sixty-nine who were surveyed did not consider themselves "old-aged" but merely "middle-aged."[31] The new trend may force us to rethink the concept of old age.

Prosperity and the tools of modern medicine mainly explain the delay of the usual ills that come in our seventies and eighties. This result appears evenly spread over North America, Japan, and Europe. As Vaupel concludes, "Most people in richer countries ... can look forward to long, healthy lives. This is arguably the most important achievement of modern civilization."[32]

In the next chapter, I explore the implications of Vaupel's finding and clear up any confusions about what extending longevity means.

NOTES

1. Jason Epstein, "The World's Oldest Living Humans." www.recordholders.org/en/list/oldest.html . See also Bernard Jeune and James W Vaupel, *Validation of Exceptional Longevity, Odense Monographs on Population Aging* Vol. 6, University Press of Southern Denmark, 1999 (English).

2. "List of Verified Oldest People," Wikepedia. http://en.wikipedia.org/wiki/List_of_the_oldest_people. *Guinness World Records 2008*, Hit Publications.

3. Jesse Green, "What Do a Bunch of Old Jews Know about Living Forever?" *New York Magazine*, November 14, 2011, 28-33, 96-98.

4. Andrew Pollack, "A Blood Test May Offer Aging Clues," *New York Times*, May 19, 2011, B1.

5. National Center for Health Statistics. www.cdc.gov/nchs/data/nvr56/nvr56_07.pdf

6. U.S. Census Bureau, International Data Base, "Total Midyear Population for the World: 1950–2050." http://www.census.gov/ipc/www/idb/worldpo html

7. "Life Expectancy and Mortality," Centers for Disease Control, *Health, United States, 2007, with Chartbook on Trends and Health of Americans*, 8. http://www.cdc.gov/nchs/data/hus/hus07.pdf#027. See also Mike Stobbe, "US Life Expectancy tops 78 for First Time," Associated Press, *Birmingham News*, June 12, 2008, A3.

8. Adding 3.5 years to those over age 50 and 2.5 years per decade after 2004.

9. Leonard Hayflick, "The Limited in vitro Lifetime of Human Diploid Cell Strains. *Experimental Cell Research* 37 (1965), 614–36.

10. Nicholas Wade, "Cancer Fighter Exacts a Price: Cellular Aging," *New York Times*, January 8, 2002, D1.

11. Trygve Tollefsbol, quoted in "The Building Blocks of Death, by Kathleen Yount, *UAB Magazine*, Spring 2008, 17. Also, personal communication of T. Tollefsbol to author, January 31, 2012.

12. Leonard Hayflick, review of *The Quest for Immortality*, by S. Olshansky, in *Radiation Research* 156 (2001), 334.

13. Gina Kolata, *Clone: The Path to Dolly, and Road Ahead*, New York, Harper, 1998.

14. Nicholas Wade, "Lives for Obese Mice, with Hope for Humans of All Sizes," *New York Times*, August 19, 2011, A1; "Prospect of Delaying Aging Ills is Raised in Cell Study in Mice," November 3, 2011, A1.

15. Ronald Bailey, *Liberation Biology, 46.*

16. Nicholas Wade, "Longevity Research Raises Hopes and Questions," *New York Times*, September 22, 2011, A19.

17. Jay Olshansky, quoted by Ron Bailey in "Forever Young," *Reason*, August/September 2002. http://reason.com/archives/2002/08/01/forever-young/singlepage

18. Oliver Wendell Holmes, "The Deacon's Masterpiece or, the Wonderful 'One-hoss Shay': A Logical Story."

> Have you heard of the wonderful one-horse shay,
> That was built in such a logical way.
> It ran a hundred years to a day,
> And then, of a sudden, it — ah, but stay,
> . . . The poor old chaise in a heap or mound
> As if it had been to the mill and ground!
> You see, of course, if you're not a dunce,
> How it went to pieces all at once,

—All at once, and nothing first,
Just as bubbles do when they burst.

19. J. E. Graham et al, "Dynamics of Cognitive Aging: Distinguishing Functional Age and Disease from Chronologic Age in a Population," *American Journal of Epidemiology* 150 (1999), 1045–54.

20. "Preventive Gerontology: Strategies for Optimizing Health Across the Life Span," *Principles of Geriatric Medicine and Gerontology*, ed. N. Honza et al., McGraw-Hill, 2003, 90. See also Robert Kane et al., *Essentials of Clinical Geriatrics*, 5th ed. McGraw-Hill, 2004, 54–55.

21. Robert Weinberg and Anthony Komaroof, "Your Lifestyle, Your Genes, and Cancer," *Newsweek*, June 23, 2008, 41–43.

22. Rand Corporation Report, "Health, Marriage, and Longer Life for Men," 1998. http://www.rand.org/pubs/research_briefs/RB5018/index1.html. Lee A. Lillard and Constantijn W.A. Panis, "Marital Status and Mortality: The Role of Health," *Demography*, 33, no. 3 (1996), 313–27; H. Liuand and D.J. Umberson, "The times they are a changin': Marital status and health differentials from 1972 to 2003," *Journal of Health and Social Behavior* 49, no. 3, 2008.

23. J. K. Petrella et al, "Potent Myofiber Hypertrophy During Resistance Training in Humans is Associated with Satellite Cell-Mediated Myonuclear Addition: A Cluster Analysis," *Journal of Applied Physiology* 1, April 2008.

24. Matt Windsor, quoting Marcus Bamman in "Strong Medicine: Prescription for a Better Life," *UAB Magazine*, Spring 2008, 13. Also, personal communication to author from Marcus Bamman, January 31, 2012.

25. Matt Windsor, quoting Marcus Bamman in "Strong Medicine: Prescription for a Better Life," *UAB Magazine*, Spring 2008, 13. See also D.J. Kosek and M. M. Bamman, "Modulation of the dystrophin-associated protein complex in response to resistance training in young and older men," *Journal of Applied Physiology* 104, no. 5, May 2008, 1476–84.

26. Mark Schoofs and Ron Winslow, "Just Sitting Back to Get in Shape: Two Pills Do the Work of Exercise," *Wall Street Journal*, August 1, 2008, A1.

27. Francis S. Collins, "Genetic Enhancements: Current and Future Prospects," December 13, 2002. Transcripts, President's Council on Bioethics.

28. James Vaupel, "Biodemography of Human Ageing," *Nature*, 464, 25 March 2010, 536–42.

29. James Vaupel, "Biodemography of Human Ageing," 536.

30. James Vaupel, "Biodemography of Human Ageing," 536.

31. National Council on Aging, Press Release, "Nearly Half of Older Americans Say, 'These Are Best Years Of My Life, National Survey Shows," March 29, 2010. http://www.ncoa.org/content.cfm?sectionID=105&detail=43

32. James Vaupel, "Biodemography of Human Ageing," 537.

Chapter Eight

Is It Wrong to Live to One Hundred?

I now want to consider some philosophical concerns about increases in human longevity. My first task is to clarify different claims. One philosophical issue involves increased longevity versus immortality. The late English philosopher Bernard Williams argued that immortal human lives would be tedious, worse than mortal lives, and meaningless.[1] Williams thinks that doing projects gives one's life meaning and that unlimited years would allow completion of all projects. Moreover, the fact that our lives end was important to him: death orders our priorities and forces us to make choices. Moreover, heroes make the ultimate choice and give up their lives to save others. If no one died, this kind of courage would be impossible.

However, for such a good philosopher, Williams made (what are often called) "category mistakes" in his essay. First, it's a jump of categories from extending life to obtaining immortality. Second, we should distinguish between *involuntary* immortality and voluntary immortality. With the latter, you can always choose—if life gets too boring—to end your life. Only the former is a sentence. Third, increased longevity involves different kinds of goals: curing aging-related diseases, increasing average life spans, curing aging itself, and obtaining voluntary immortality. We shouldn't conflate these.

So let's try to drill down to more basic philosophical claims. Let's assume we won't be immortal soon, that we won't cure aging at the cellular level (because of the Hayflick limit), and that any increase in longevity would be voluntary, such that, if life got too tedious, it could always be ended.

If James Vaupel is correct, then the incremental enhancements that have been ongoing over the last decades have extended morbidity and mortality accordion-like by at least a decade for healthy people in developed countries. If so, Bismarck's age of sixty-five for being old and retired may need to be extended to seventy-five—in other words, "seventy-five is the new sixty-five."

Assuming the trend spotted by James Vaupel is correct, is it a good thing? To some impatient people, the question is stupid. Why wouldn't anyone want to live more rather than less? Well, another view exists here, with some cogent objections, but we need to carefully separate its claims.

One claim is that extended life is a *misguided use of resources*. Bioethicist Daniel Callahan of the Hastings Institute, who was born in 1930, opposes research to extend life.[2] He thinks we should accept our present life span, not invest in research to extend old age. Or to be more precise, he argues that wise people should have better ways to spend their monies on research than extending human lives. Social conservative Leon Kass, born in 1939, also seems to claim that trying to extend human life foolishly wastes resources.

This objection now seems moot. As said, various enrichments have combined to allow healthy people to live longer, including ones not previously mentioned, such as fluoridated water, statins to reduce inflammation and the effects of cholesterol, assisted living in group homes, better nutrition, physical therapy after injuries, better dental care, good public transportation, and efficient departments of public health. These improvements *both* improved the quality of existing lives *and* thereby extended longevity. Extending longevity never was an either/or choice.

Another objection is that extending life is *not natural*. To rebut this claim, recall the figures about human longevity that began this chapter. Which expected human longevity is natural? Death in ancient Sparta by age thirty-five? Death in 1900 in America at age forty-seven? For those now living, death by age ninety-five? If the human life span peaks at

125, why is death at any point along the spectrum more natural than any other? Moreover, if fifty years of life is good, why isn't one hundred?

If we could enter a time machine and switch lives with someone in 1900, few people would just want to live to the then-predicted life expectancy of forty-seven years. Parents would not understand what is wrong with living to eighty-four rather than to forty-seven. We don't believe, as anti-aging researchers such as Francis Fukuyama imply, that a newborn girl who lives an extra thirty-seven years might lose her humanity and become "post-human."[3] What is natural is relative to what century one is born into.

Another objection might be that extending human life is *foolish*. Why, cynics ask, will people want to live so long? Won't people become sad? Suppose you outlive your parents, your siblings, and your good friends. Maybe you outlive your children. Wouldn't it be sad to be alone and so old? Maybe you were foolish to want to live so long.

An associated view of Callahan and Kass, abetted lately by Yale surgeon-essayist Sherwin Nuland, is that society wastes a lot of money in the last year of life pursuing a lousy last few months of life. *New York Times* essayist David Brooks recently uncritically accepted this falsehood.[4]

But the great logical fallacy here is to only calculate the cost of the last year of life *for those patients who actually died*. What about the other 80 percent who recovered, went home to live another five years with their families, and who were quite glad to have had the money spent on them for their recoveries? If you want to do a fair study, take a group of one hundred eighty-five-year-olds in a hospital and calculate how much is spent on them for twelve months. Then compare the costs for those who died during that year with the costs of those who lived. Then, for those who lived, prorate the costs over their new years of living.

But not everyone sees extra years of living, like Callahan-Kass-Nuland-Brooks, as years of misery. For starters, maybe everyone you know would also live a nice long life, including your children and friends. Michael Kinsley wrote in 2008 in the *New Yorker* about "the biggest competition of all."

Ask yourself: what do you have now, and what do you covet, that you would not gladly trade for, say, five extra years? These would be good years, of cross-country skiing between fashionable Colorado resorts, or at least years when you could still walk and think and read and drive.[5]

As Kinsley points out, "Life would be pretty empty without your friends. But not as empty as death." Sure, you may be lonely, but you can also make new friends.

Are these shallow personal values? Kinsley also ridicules the "shallow" idea that "he who dies with the most toys, wins," noting that lust for longevity trumps because "what good are toys if you're dead? 'He Who Dies Last'— he's the one who wins."

One thing they could also mean is that it will be *boring* to live longer. Perhaps that will be true for some people.

However, a survey of life over the last fifty years reveals that various advances helped (what Tom Brokaw famously called) "the Greatest Generation" live twenty more years of high-quality life than their parents. For my parents (both of whom made it into their late eighties), their last two decades differed little in quality and functionality from their own parents' last two decades, *but they had an additional twenty years of good living.* The Study of Adult Development at Harvard University, the longest study over decades ever conducted, falsified the view that as they get older, men turn into curmudgeons. Instead, men got happier as they got older.[6] Another 2011 study, which followed two large groups of Boston-area men, found that men became happier in their sixties and seventies, not crabby and depressed.[7]

One member of this greatest generation, Corporal Frank Buckles, lied at age sixteen to enlist in the army and to see action in World War I.[8] He lived robustly for 110 years and until he died in 2011, he was our oldest living veteran. Each morning, he did fifty sit-ups, lifted two-pound weights, and stretched major groups of muscles. Buckles remained so mentally alert that, at age 106, he stated in 2007 that the United States should only go to war when it's an emergency, and implied then that invading Iraq was not such an emergency.[9] *Because* of his nearly eleven decades, not *despite* them, Frank Buckles lived well and wisely.

"We've entered a new age of old age," said James Firman, president and CEO of the National Council on Aging. "The possibility of experiencing positive, vital aging lasting into our tenth decade of life is one of the new realities of the 21st century."[10]

But if you live an extra twenty years, isn't that selfish? Think of all the resources you're consuming! Well, not necessarily. The longer you live, the more you care about the future. It's one thing to burn down the savannah to hunt game if you're starving; it's quite another if you plan to live to one hundred. Taking it one step further, people who expected to live two hundred years would care much more about environmental pollution and the integrity of the world's financial system because they would have a greater stake in what happens.

Also, the longer we expect to live, the greater our motivation to save. This might revive the dying virtue of saving money, as compound interest would build up much more over a hundred years than seventy.

With an average life of 105 rather than 85, one might pursue not one, but three careers—perhaps one as a Navy medic, one as a bioethicist, and one as a travel guide. You would cultivate a different set of virtues in the extra thirty years, but not the present ones of old age that center on frailty, physicians, and hospitals.

Within a life, one way to view two extra decades (or even two extra centuries) is as a neutral tool, neither good nor bad in itself. Like any tool, different people may use it differently. A hammer can be used to build a house or to kill humans. Some people will use a new tool wisely, others foolishly. If someone has made bad choices, then the extra decades will make them worse, but others, who make good choices, can enjoy the benefits.

A third philosophical issue raised by two more decades of life concerns relationships to members of one's family. This is a complex issue.

If the *average* woman lives a century, this will create what Wittgenstein called a different "form of life," especially from her ancestors, where in 1900 the same woman would have only lived to fifty. It is as if a person gets to live twice, in two different worlds, while retaining the same self.

Many relationships within a family evolved from past practices. In developing countries without old age safety nets such as Social Security and Medicare in the United States, having children to care for you is essential. This is one reason why families in India and China have lots of children and value boys more, as males are obligated to care for their parents.

In developed countries, different gender obligations have prevailed. Females more often care for parents of their own and their husband's. Such "sandwich" women may both raise their own children and care for aging parents and in-laws. The downside of living a century is that a caring woman could get burdened with caring for too many people: her children, her parents, and some grandparents too.

In this context, philosopher Jane English famously raised the question, "What Do Grown Children Owe their Parents?"[11] Here the "owe" means "what parents can claim from grown children *as their right*." For English, children and parents over decades should become friends and children ideally should care for parents out of love. But if they are not friends and no love exists, grown children are not obligated to provide for their parents. Simply because their parents brought them into the world and raised them does not create such an obligation in part because children had no choice in the matter.

Although technically her arguments may be valid, the feelings that exist within families do not run along valid arguments. I expect that, as people live longer, families will need to negotiate new arrangements. Some senior citizens will fear being burdens and insure that they are not. Others won't be so organized.

Tennessee philosopher John Hardwig famously argued that seniors in some circumstances should not ask their middle-aged children to sacrifice for them.[12] English's and Hardwig's pieces should be considered opening salvos in a new intergenerational war about resources owed to those over age seventy.

Another issue to consider is work. Vaupel wonders whether the nature of work may need restructuring to accommodate so many people living so long. Using the example of Germany, he speculates that this country, if more people work longer, may need to reduce the average workweek so that more people can work.

Japan seems to be facing this problem now, with much of advanced Europe close behind.[13] Japan has too many people over eighty and too many financially secure people aged fifty to seventy. The latter stay so long in their careers that they hog all the good jobs in education, business, and professions. Most twenty- to thirty-year-old Japanese believe they face a closed future and that they must leave Japan to find real opportunities to advance.

Consider also tenure in teaching in K–12 education and in universities. It is one thing to tenure a teacher for twenty-five years, but another for forty or fifty. How many teachers can retain their enthusiasm for such a period? How many professors? As education downsizes and tenured spots become a scarce resource, can an efficient society bestow sinecures that might last for five decades?

A fourth philosophical issue involves justice. Some might object that, unless we increase longevity for everyone, extra life in developed countries would create global resentment, so none should have it until all can have it. Can we really justify, critics ask, a medical world where rich people in Europe and North America live three times longer *on average* than the poorest people in Botswana?

First, there's little that short-lived people can do about others living longer because *it's not as if the years are transferable.* Second, longevity will be a symptom of inequality, not a cause of it. Finally, the masses of the world are unlikely to rise up against citizens of developed countries merely because the latter live longer. Already, although the average life span in Botswana is thirty-four and eighty-four in Japan, you don't see dying Botswanans protesting the long lives of Japanese.

It is also true that not everyone will live longer. Until we find a cure for cancer, coronary artery disease, and stroke, these three diseases will be the cause of death for most people before age eighty. If they don't succumb to these three, aging at the cellular level will weaken the immune system, making those over eighty vulnerable to other diseases. Even if we cured these major diseases, we're not safe yet. Of the 2.4 million Americans who died in 2001, about 13,000 died from bites and poisons, another 13,000 died from falls, about 44,000 died in automobile crashes, and firearms figured in another 30,000 deaths. [14] If none of these get you, doctors and hospitals may: according to the Institute of Medicine, mistakes by medical personnel kill nearly one hundred thousand Americans each year. [15]

Despite all these dangers waiting to kill us, more and more of us will live until our eighties and nineties. More and more will become centenarians, especially those born today in middle-class families with good medical and dental coverage. By 1990, about 37,000 Americans lived to be over one hundred years old, yet by 2050, according to the National Institute on Aging, four million will live to become centenarians. [16]

But can an advanced society *afford* for us to live these extra years? The philosophical issue here is not about global, but rather, domestic justice. If senior Americans live too long, won't they consume too many resources, resources that might otherwise be given to young Americans? This argument stings: "Die early, so younger people can get your money." Will intergenerational war soon divide young against old? Has it already started?

Past projections about Medicare, social security, life insurance, long-term care insurance, annuities, mortgages, and savings assume a normal human life span. Already citizens in developed countries live far longer than the life envisioned by the founders of our old-age systems.

In Bismarck's time, most people did not make it to fifty, much less sixty-five, so few resources were needed to fund his pension. When Social Security began in 1935, only about half of men and about two thirds of women lived to age sixty-five, and for them, at retirement they could expect to live eleven more years. Today, about three-fourths of men and nearly 85 percent of women live to that age and can expect to live another sixteen years.

The savings of past workers do not fund Social Security and Medicare, but taxes from current workers. It's a revolving-door system of financing, where current workers pay for benefits of existing senior citizens. Decades ago, about two workers paid for every beneficiary receiving Social Security or Medicare. As Baby Boomers retire, things could get bad, with two people benefiting for every worker taxed. Obviously, the amount of taxes has to rise, the number of beneficiaries has to shrink, or the amount of benefits has to fall.

Worse, many states have made commitments to retirees, both for pensions and medical coverage, that they have not funded; these commitments depend on the trust and goodwill of future taxpayers of that state, but such taxpayers may have never voted for such payments. Is a generational war brewing? In 2050, will workers under age seventy be taxed at 60 percent of earnings to pay for entitlements of long-living, retired Americans?

We could mitigate this problem. Although the United States pays for Social Security and Medicare by taxing working citizens, adjustments can keep the system operating. The age when one can first withdraw Social Security can be raised. This is like a tax on current workers, so if they must feel pain, so must others. Benefits to current retirees can be reduced, while taxes on the youngest and healthiest can be increased. To make the system just and functional, everybody should sacrifice something.[17]

More radically, illegal working immigrants could legally be allowed to stay in the country on the condition that they pay twice as much as other Americans into FICA and the Medicare Trust Fund (it's only "unfair" if they refuse the bargain and for most, *legal* entry on these terms would be better than not being able to enter or remaining illegal immigrants).

Third, more immigrants want to enter the United States, thereby growing the work force and increasing the number of taxpayers. Fourth, the U.S. population itself is expanding. Just a few decades ago it was at 200 million; in 2007, it topped 300 million. That's a lot of extra tax-paying workers.

In the debate over reforming Medicare in 2011, one Republican senator claimed that the average beneficiary of Medicare paid in $150,000 and gets $350,000 in benefits. If we allow millions of Americans to draw an extra twenty years of Medicare benefits, younger workers will be financially crushed.

From the point of view of the tragedy of the commons and intergenerational justice, it is obviously unfair that one generation might be able to use up so many resources at the expense of another. Whether that last phrase is true is the big question, i.e., whether the Baby Boomers living longer and better will be at the expense of Generation X living shorter and worse.

For me, it is going to be hard not to use up expensive medical resources, especially for the abstract goal of helping younger workers. But I hate to think my living longer is an injustice to my students and their generation. To avoid this, we should plan for what is coming.

NOTES

1. Bernard Williams, "The Makropoulos Case: Reflections on the Tedium of Immortality," in his *Problems of the Self* (Cambridge: Cambridge University Press, 1973).

2. Daniel Callahan, *What Kind of Life? The Limits of Medical Progress* (New York, Simon & Schuster, 1990).

3. Fukuyama, Francis, *Our Posthuman Future: Consequences of the Biotechnology Revolution* (New York: Farrar, Straus & Giroux, 2002).

4. David Brooks, "Death and Budgets," *New York Times*, July 14, 2011.

5. Michael Kinsley, "Mine is Longer than Yours," *New Yorker*, April 7, 2008, 38ff.

6. Laboratory of Adult Development, Harvard University, http://adultdev.bwh.harvard.edu/research-SAD.html

7. Christine Stapleton, "Study: Men Get Happier as They Age," *Cincinnati Enquirer* and Cox News Service, March 3, 2011, E2.

8. http://en.wikipedia.org/wiki/Frank_Buckles

9. "106-year-old WWI Veteran Speaks on Iraq War," *Washington Post*, November 12, 2007.

10. "106-year-old WWI Veteran Speaks on Iraq War."

11. Jane English, "What Do Grown Children Owe Their Parents?" *Philosophical and Legal Reflections on Parenthood*, Onora O'Neill and William Ruddick, eds. (New York: Oxford, 1979).

12. John Hardwig, "Is There A Duty to Die?" *Hastings Center Report*, 27, no. 2 (1997): 34–42.

13. Martin Flackler, *New York Times*, January 27, 2011, "In Japan, Young Face Generational Roadblocks."

14. *National Vital Statistics Report*, Vol. 15, September 16, 2002.

15. Institute of Medicine, *To Err is Human: Building a Safer Health System*, (eds) Linda T. Kohn, et al., Committee on Quality of Health Care in America (Washington, D.C.: National Academy Press, 2000).

16. Jesse Green, "What Do a Bunch of Old Jews Know about Living Forever?" *New York Magazine*, November 14, 2011, 31.

17. This was what the UAB Ethics Bowl Team argued in winning its case in the 2011 regional competition in Tampa about precisely this kind of case.

Chapter Nine

A Better Life with Personalized Genetics

In this chapter, I consider the modest project of understanding one's own genome and how this might affect one's future health. This is essentially a self-regarding project.

The press has reported extensively about personalized analysis of one's genes to predict future genetic diseases. One day, we may use such analyses to forestall expression of our gene-based diseases. Indeed, a continuum exists where genetic testing might benefit a particular individual to the other extreme, where it might be harmful. In an ideal case, an analysis of one's personal genotype and its minute variations might be correlated with how well medicines work for one's genotype and predict one's future risks. As I will explain, all of that will be tricky and complex.

Some clear-cut cases exist where individuals will benefit from self-testing. Consider David Bloom, an NBC television reporter who went to Iraq in 2003 to cover the war. He didn't know he carried a genetic disorder prevalent in 2–7 percent of Caucasians, Factor V Leiden, the most common clotting disorder among Americans. It placed him at high risk for a lethal blood clot. [1]

Had Bloom known, he might not have taken long plane flights, ridden on military vehicles in tight spaces that hurt his circulation, or lived in dehydrating environments. Because he had Factor V Leiden, all of these elements combined to create the blood clot that lodged in Bloom's lungs and killed him.

Prior to 2008, Americans might have been reluctant to test themselves for genetic disorders for fear either of losing their medical coverage or not being able to buy life insurance. The Genetic Information Non Discrimination Act (GINA) now protects them against such dangers.[2]

Genetic tests are becoming cheaper and more comprehensive. Cases like Bloom's, along with GINA, give people a reason to test. As of 2009, several U.S. companies offered such tests. They use mail-in swabs taken from scrapes inside the cheek, a method of testing dubbed "spit genomics."

Because it identifies both good and bad conditions, personalized genetic testing is the ultimate double-edged sword. To see this, consider the story of clinical psychologist Nancy Wexler, who for decades taught clinical neuropsychology at Columbia University.

After Wexler's mother died of Huntington's disease, a devastating neurological disease lacking treatment, she embarked on a quest to find the Huntington's gene. Because the gene is autosomal dominant, Nancy and her sister Alice each had a 50 percent risk of inheriting it. Because the average age of onset is thirty-six, female victims often bear children before learning they are affected. At present, 25,000 Americans have it and about 100,000 Americans have an afflicted parent.

In 1986, before personalized genetic testing was available, Wexler worked for ten years to develop a test so that she could take it. However, when a test did become available in the 1990s, she famously changed her mind and decided *not* to take it. The implications of her decision stunned people in medical genetics. A leading advocate for testing who carried a 50 percent risk, had decided not to find out if she had the gene.

Moreover, she was a clinical psychologist who should've known herself. Indeed, not only did Wexler not take the test, she became an advocate for *not* taking it. What happened? It turned out to be something important psychologically.

Wexler decided she had nothing to gain by taking the test. If she had the disease, it was fully penetrant, meaning that she would eventually lose her mind to it. If she did not have it, well, that would be great.

But what if she had the gene and it didn't start penetrating for two decades? Could she live with that knowledge? "Once you get that kind of knowledge," she said, "you can't take it back."

In other words, the predictive knowledge might be toxic, creating a sense of impending doom. To people who want to be tested before they go to law school, she says: "Go to law school! Develop your mind! What are you going to do if you're positive? Spend the rest of your life waiting to be a patient?"

As Wexler's story shows, the main risk of early presymptomatic testing is *developing a sick identity*. Can someone thrive, knowing she has a ticking time bomb inside her for ovarian cancer, cystic fibrosis, or sickle cell disease? Will self-diagnosed people spend the rest of their lives *waiting to get sick*?

This will be true for suggestible people. And some of us may turn out to be more suggestible than we think.

The 1997 movie *GATTACA* influenced many people who wrongly concluded that its message was that willpower can triumph over genes or that nurture is just as important as nature. But its real message was that being labeled genetically defective or superior can be self-fulfilling.

In the movie, the genetically superior son, Jerome, to whom the father is proud to give his name, feels superior to the naturally conceived son, Vincent. While swimming in the ocean as adults, Jerome one day loses a game of chicken to Vincent, and suddenly Jerome's self-confidence collapses. Because his superiority had not been earned, Jerome had not built up the necessary virtues to cope with any loss to Vincent.

On the other hand, Vincent had struggled for any tidbit of recognition from his prejudiced father or his worried mother. Always afraid that he will hurt himself or get sick, his mother won't let him do anything. He can't attend good schools because he has been labeled a health risk and the schools can't afford to insure him. However, Vincent's inner resources exceed Jerome's, for everything Vincent has achieved has been through fierce effort, self-modification, and lofty aspirations.

In one of the most famous studies in psychiatry, the 1973 Rosenhan study, various health professionals, including psychiatrists, pretended to be paranoid schizophrenics and had themselves committed to a mental institution.[3] Once labeled as such, the staff treated the psychiatrists as real, paranoid schizophrenics. When they dropped their act and told the staff who they really were, the staff refused to believe them ("Oh, really? You're the Chief of Psychiatry at Harvard? Right!").

Potent is the effect of being labeled, either by medical professionals or by parents, either as gifted or as retarded. Tests that bring such labels immediately influence parents, siblings, your own sense of self, and future employers. Similar results occur when labels drop on you for being diabetic, gay, alcoholic, heart-defective, or a good sprinter.

The Rosenhan study, the story of Nancy Wexler, and the message of *GATTACA* suggest that we should be careful about taking presymptomatic genetic tests. If a test for prostate cancer has only a 50 percent rate of accuracy, we should avoid it. If a positive test might lead a man to confuse benign prostate enlargement with initial symptoms of real cancer, or worse, to fret about every twitch and spasm, he should avoid it.

In 2008, journalists ran a spate of articles about testing small kids for sports genes such as ACTN3, a gene supposedly correlated to superb athletes.[4] While the R variant of the ACTN3 gene makes bodies produce alpha-actinin-3, a protein found in fast-twitch muscles, the X variant inhibits production. In one Australian study, 50 percent of elite white sprinters had two copies of the R variant, and all male Olympians in power sports had a least one copy. On the other hand, the X variant supposedly makes people more suitable for endurance sports such as cross-country running. Top endurance athletes are somewhat more likely than normal to have two copies of the X variant than a control group (25 percent to 18 percent), and no elite female sprinter had two copies of the X variant.

Australian company Genetic Technologies offers this test in North America through a company called Atlas and its Web site.[5] For $150 parents and coaches can swab inside a child's cheek to discover what kind of muscles a child will develop. In a pyramidical system such as China's, designed to identify young athletes with potential and support their development, such testing will be another tool to select those for maximal coaching.

These tests seem prime candidates for the dangers of labeling. If a kid tests positive for the R variant, he will be labeled a sprinter (and not a mathematician or essayist). Worse, if he lacks the ACTN3 gene, his athletic parents might sigh and say, "Alas, you're only going to be a mathematician or essayist!"

What about testing yourself in personalized genomics for diabetes? Diabetes might be a disease where it makes sense to take a presymptomatic test. Uncontrolled, it leads to very bad results: kidney failure, retinal damage (which can lead to blindness), gangrene (especially in legs, leading to amputation), damage to nerves, and heart failure. In 2006, scientists at DeCode Genetics discovered a gene for Type 2 diabetes. People who get two copies of the gene from their parents have twice the likelihood of developing diabetes as those who don't carry any copies. Being born with one copy raises the risk above average by 40 percent (about 38 percent of Northern Europeans, as well as many African Americans, carry one copy.) Seven percent of these groups carry two copies and thus have a whopping 140 percent increase in risk.[6] Presumably, Far Eastern Asians carry a similar gene, explaining the incidence of diabetes in this population when they migrate to developed countries.

In 2006, epidemiologists discovered an epidemic of Type 2 diabetes in New York City. Over 800,000 of its citizens, more than 1 in 8, had Type 2 diabetes.[7] This incidence is one-third higher than that of the nation. In East Harlem, as many as one in five people have this kind of diabetes.[8]

Type 2 diabetes is an especially good candidate for prevention because we know that many Asian people do not get diabetes until they adopt Western lifestyles. If we could presymptomatically test young people for genes for diabetes, we could urge people with two copies to be especially careful about their diets.

Consumers need to understand that most information from genetic tests will NOT be given like this: "You have a gene for Alzheimer's disease and you lack genes for breast and colon cancer." Instead, the information will look like: "Given your ethnicity and gender, and because you have one copy of a gene for Type 2 diabetes, your chances of having diabetes are 40 percent greater than other members of your ethnicity and gender."

Note that in talking about genes, we need to distinguish between *absolute and relative risk*. If the absolute risk of diabetes is low, say, as is Type 2 diabetes in Africa, then having one or two copies of this new gene doesn't mean that huge numbers of Africans will get diabetes. As a 2009 survey of prediction of risk of disease from genetics remarked, "The great majority of the newly identified risk-marker alleles confer very small relative risks, ranging from 1.1 to 1.5."[9]

The standard view in public health is that Type 2 diabetes "can be delayed and perhaps prevented with changes in diet and exercise. Although both types are believed to stem in part from genetic factors, Type 2 is also spurred by obesity and inactivity."[10]

But given our discussion of the power of belief in genetic reductionism, labeling, and sick identities, how many people tested might reconceptualize themselves as diabetics –long before they had any symptoms? Would such a description become their identity?

Given all these factors, do you take a screening test for cancer, diabetes, and Alzheimer's? Here we come to an important divide about taking genetic tests and risking bad news. Two recent studies of presymptomatic testing for Alzheimer's found that some people getting bad news report not feeling devastated.[11]

On the other hand, some people can't imagine hearing bad news and take the attitude of, "If there's no treatment for a terrible gene-based disease, why test for it in advance?" But according to the authors of these studies, only a minority of respondents didn't want to know their results, and if this minority didn't, it was because they didn't want to live knowing they had Alzheimer's in their future.

After I wrote a nationally-circulated op-ed expressing these views,[12] *Reason* magazine's science editor, Ron Bailey, disagreed, writing that "bioethicists Can't Handle the Truth."[13] The pun on Jack Nicholson's character in *A Few Good Men* resonates well, because those who want the truth and who want others to get theirs generally take what Nancy Wexler calls "a macho attitude" to truth-telling. Time will tell if they are as macho as they seem when they discover they've inherited a fatal genetic disease.

Here it seems that some people just want to know—indeed, *must* know—what can be known. Others feel just as strongly the opposite way. At this point, all anyone can say is, "To each his own." So long as people are informed, each person has the right to find out all he can about his gene-based future. In this way, it's like reading a lot about taking modafinil or undergoing cosmetic surgery, and then going ahead and taking the drug or having the surgery.

In discussing previous enhancements, I discussed snake oil salesmen in enhancement medicine and emphasized that understanding issues in bioethics requires following the money trail. Genetic self-testing is one such perilous area because millions of people may pay $500 to a $1,000 to test themselves for a genetic disease but waste their money. Why?

In 2002, Myriad Genetics of Salt Lake City expanded its sales force from 85 to 600 agents to market BRCA1 testing directly to doctors and their patients. The tests, which cost between $750 and $2,750, would only benefit the 5 to 10 percent of people with breast cancer caused by these genes.

Mass marketing of such a test is a win-win situation for Myriad Genetics. For the people who test positive, they get their money's worth and advance news. For the people who test negative, they get relief and will not complain about the money spent. The ethical issue arises when thousands of people seek relief by genetic self-testing who are really not at genetic risk: they waste their money to get a negative result. But perhaps it's patronizing to say they shouldn't waste their money as they want.

Similar tests are now offered for genes for prostate cancer and fast-twitch muscles of superior athletes, only a small percentage of which is caused by a single gene. For most people, such testing will waste their money.

Almost every month, the mass media report the discovery of an alleged gene for a disease or a trait, for example, for humor. Yet almost all such reports mislead us into thinking the genetic revolution has come. In fact, when we look for applications in ordinary medicine, we see the reality: progress is slow, hesitant, and results come with many qualifications.

Some people act radically on new genetic information. Some patients, when they discover they carry genes for breast or ovarian cancer, get double mastectomies or ovarectomies. Bioethicist Art Caplan tells the story of a parent at a genetics clinic at the University of Pennsylvania who wanted to test his eleven-year-old daughter for breast cancer genes and, if she were positive, do preventive mastectomies.[14]

Like eugenics, much of the news about genetics in today's mass media is simplistic, alarmist, and premature. The movie *GATTACA* dramatizes both genetic fatalism and the dangers of labeling. Many companies will try to sell you genetic testing; if you do buy, caveat emptor, and be sure the news doesn't doom you to your spouse, parents, friends, or self with a toxic label.

One final lesson about caveat emptor: David Agus, a professor of medicine and engineering at the University of Southern California, cofounded two personalized medicine companies, Navigenics and Applied Proteomics. His *The End of Illness* prophesizes that, from a drop of your blood, companies will tell you whether to take a new drug to lower your risk of cancer, stop the expression of a lethal genetic package, or spot drug interactions.[15] As well, they will monitor your life every day via Google, Smartphones, and social media. But beware anyone like Agus selling you stock in his companies or asking you to buy his products. Where is he going to get his data? Agus says in an op-ed, "What is equally exciting is that this patient data will be added to a universal database that can be aggregated by powerful search engines like Google and constantly fed into new trials and experiments..."[16]

No way! Google's attempt to have us put our medical records in its safekeeping failed miserably because no one trusted its commitment to privacy. This claim will fail for similar reasons. Insurance companies seek information on those with newly diagnosed heart conditions and won't want to insure them. Why would savvy consumers share such information with Google when it is selling their information to for-profit companies?

More fundamentally to the project of Agus, for personalized medicine to work, millions of us would need to sign up for randomized clinical trials to prove that having x, y, and z genes, and then doing A, B, or C, led to a longer, better life. Without such studies, it's all speculation, and I don't see many of us rushing to join such studies or anyone rushing to fund them.

In conclusion, the message of this chapter is mixed: genetic testing could have saved David Bloom's life. For some highly competent, highly motivated people, such testing may help them stave off cancer or diabetes. For many others, such testing may give them a genetic burden they wish they never had to know. For most, it will be a waste of money.

NOTES

1. "Disorder Magnifies Blood Clot Risk," Jane Brody, *New York Times*, June 10, 2008, D7.

2. National Human Genome Research Institute, "Fact Sheet on the Genetic Information Nondiscrimination Act (GINA) of 2008. http://www.genome.gov/24519851 (accessed 1/10/2012).

3. D. L. Rosenhan "On Being Sane in Insane Places." *Science* 179 (January 1973), 250–58.

4. Juliet Macur, "Born to Run? Little Ones Get Test for Sports Gene," *New York Times*, November 30, 2008.

5. http://www.atlasgene.com/

6. "Diabetes Gene Detected," *Sydney Morning Herald*, January 19, 2006.
7. N. R. Kleinfield, "Diabetes and Its Awful Toll," *New York Times*, January 9, 2006.
8. N. R. Kleinfield, "Living at the Epicenter of Diabetes, Defiance and Despair," *New York Times*, January 10, 2006.
9. Peter Kraft et. al., "Genetic Risk Prediction—Are We There Yet?" *New England Journal of Medicine* 23 April 2009, 360, no. 17, 1701.
10. N. R. Kleinfield, "Diabetes and Its Awful Toll."
11. R. C. Green et. al., "Disclosure of *APOE* Genotype for Risk of Alzheimer's Disease," *New England Journal of Medicine*, 2009; 361, 245–54.
12. Gregory Pence, "Should We Test for Genetic Diseases that Can't Be Cured?" *Birmingham News*, January 9, 2011.
13. Ron Bailey, "Bioethicists Can't Handle the Truth," *REASON*, February 2011.
14. http://thedianerehmshow.org/shows/2010-12-31/dna-sequencing-personal-genomics-rebroadcast/transcript
15. David Agus, *The End of Illness* (New York: Free Press, 2012).
16. David Agus, "A Doctor in Your Pocket," *Wall Street Journal*, January 14, 2012.

PART II

CHOOSING BETTER FUTURE CHILDREN

Chapter Ten

Building Better Kids: Choosing Embryos

In this book, I discuss several themes. First, Alarmists impede progress in making humans better. Second, both Alarmists and Enthusiasts focus too much on genetic interventions, which, at this point, are impractical and dangerous. Third, more practical ways than genetic intervention exist to improve humans—ways we presently ignore. The next four chapters focus on such practical ways: before birth, during gestation, at birth, and during childhood.

Although this chapter is entitled "Building Better Kids: Choosing Embryos," it could have been be entitled "How Not to Worry about Eugenics." In bioethics, the topic is commonly called "PGD," which stands for "preimplantation genetic diagnosis." PGD refers to selecting healthy embryos for use in assisted reproduction.

We should discuss the idea of choosing an embryo that is healthy and not, say, blind. Is that morally permissible? Does it discriminate against existing people with disabilities?

Many couples *choose* to be pregnant and *want* a baby, but, rightly or wrongly, don't want a baby with Down syndrome, spina bifida, or any of hundreds of congenital conditions causing life-long impairments. When given the choice, and regardless of the efforts of organizations for people with disabilities, most prospective parents choose against disability and want a "normal" baby. Unlike a typical abortion, they do not choose against continuing a pregnancy, but instead choose not to have *any* baby with a disability.

In doing so, are they stealth eugenicists? Revealing prejudice against people with disabilities? I don't think so. They are simply trying to be good parents who want the best for their children. Nothing could be more natural than such choices; nothing could more express the high hopes of all parents for future children.

Although no abortion is easy, choosing against a serious genetic disease is one of the easiest cases of abortion to justify. Not every family can handle raising a special-needs child. As a general rule, most families cherish the right to choose the number (and if they can choose, even the kind) of children who will make up their family.

Forty years ago, when geneticists developed the first crude tests that predicted genetic diseases, Alarmists such as Leon Kass warned of eugenics.[1] They have cried wolf so many times that their continued cries cause sophisticated people to yawn. Yet their effect lingers on average citizens, especially through movies such as *GATTACA* and *The Island*.

Disability advocates contend that such genetic testing of embryos creates a new eugenics and will result in massive deaths of fetuses that carry genes for undesirable conditions. First-trimester abortions account for 88 percent of abortions.[2] Anti-abortion advocates fear that genetic testing during this trimester will legitimize massive abortions.

At this point, I need to talk more about "eugenics" and its two meanings. Contrary to popular belief, eugenics did not start in Nazi Germany, but on Long Island, New York. Based on a smidgen of fact, it inferred many incorrect conclusions.

In 1859, Charles Darwin published *On the Origin of Species*, defending the evolution of humans from primates and using concepts such as competitive advantage and survival of the fittest. Because it contradicted the biblical story of creation of Adam and Eve, Darwin's book took decades for people to accept (even today, some *still* do not accept it).

In the late 1880s, Darwin's cousin Francis Galton invented "eugenics" (literally, good birth) and championed maximal births by the most "fit" people, as well as sterilization or voluntary abstinence of "unfit" people. By 1905, eugenic organizations had sprung up in Europe, Japan, and Scandinavia, but especially on Long Island. U.S. politicians and geneticists urged "eugenic marriages" and sterilization of the unfit; they worried that incoming hordes of Irish, Italian, Chinese, and African immigrants, who tended to have large families, undermined the WASP-ish "breeding stock" of America.

Because of these ideas, thirty-one states passed laws allowing involuntary sterilization of "mental defectives." By 1941, 36,000 Americans had been sterilized.[3] In Nazi Germany, Hitler gave these ideas greater power, and physicians sterilized 225,000 involuntary people in that country for perceived mental illness or perceived inheritable physical disabilities. The Immigration Restriction Act of 1924 severely limited entry into the United States of people from "inferior" lands such as Asia, Africa, southern Europe, and Ireland, while encouraging immigration from England, Germany, Switzerland, and Scandinavia.

Racism and falsehoods fueled most of the early ideas of eugenics. Early geneticists did not know that mental retardation could be caused not only by inherited conditions, but also by chromosomal breakage.[4] They did not know which human traits came from genes and which from the environment (or the interaction of both). They did not completely understand dominant and recessive genes, and the principles of population genetics, so they miscalculated how long it would take to eliminate bad genes from a population. Most egregiously, they did not understand, or care about, the degree of state coercion necessary to control reproduction in millions of people and the consequent violation of their procreative liberty. Later in the twentieth century, when China limited couples to one child, the world discovered the severity of measures needed to accomplish reproductive control of a population, for example, publicly starving or continually humiliating a couple that has two children.[5]

By 1935, the geneticist Herman J. Muller bemoaned that eugenics was "hopelessly perverted," a cult for "advocates for race and class prejudice, defenders of vested interests of church and State, Fascists, Hitlerites, and reactionaries generally."[6] Another leading geneticist of the time, and a founding father of statistical genetics, J. B. S. Haldane, said "many of the deeds done in America in the name of eugenics are about as much justified by science as were the proceedings of the Inquisition by the Gospels."[7]

After World War II, bad science and the Nazi's "Final Solution" discredited eugenics. Afterward, eugenics secretly continued in Scandinavia. In Sweden, physicians continued to forcibly sterilize citizens with low intelligence or gross physical defects until 1976.[8] Similar, secret eugenic sterilizations occurred during the same decades in China and Australia.[9] In 2011, Americans learned that about 7,000 poor black women were sterilized between 1920 and 1974 in North Carolina to reduce welfare rolls and to cleanse the gene pool of undesirable characteristics. [10]

Now we must emphasize why the past eugenics movement does not equate to increased choice today by parents against genetic disease nor to ethical attempts to enhance humans. The past eugenics movement was evil: it employed state coercion, had false views of how to eradicate genetic disease, and was racist. I call this Eugenics with a capital "E."

What opponents today decry as "eugenics" is not the movement discussed above in which some women and couples were forced to abort their fetuses or where many were sterilized. Instead, people *voluntarily* choose to abort to prevent genetic disease, based not on false information about their fetuses but upon reliable data. In Australia, for example, the number of babies born with Down syndrome to mothers younger than age thirty-five dropped by half thanks to better, earlier information. [11] I call this "eugenics" with a lower-case "e."

Is this new eugenics wrong? Critics say "yes," for two reasons. First, when couples choose against having a child with Down syndrome, they send a message to existing people with Down syndrome that their lives are not worth living and that their parents should have aborted them. Second, it devalues people with disabilities in public policy and hence, will result in fewer resources for existing people with disabilities. So the master philosophical question here is whether a just public policy can both support parents choosing against undesirable genetic conditions and also not devalue the lives of existing people with these genetic conditions.

Pioneering British bioethicist Jonathan Glover argues that "ugly attitudes" that limit the lives of people with disabilities and express contempt for them are wrong. [12] But he also argues that parents' preferences for a normal, rather than a disabled, child can co-exist with good attitudes.

For Glover, people can believe that first, people with disabilities have rewarding lives, that parenting children with disabilities can make families happy, and that society should provide resources for such parents and children to flourish, and second, they can still prefer to raise normal children. Just as some parents delay conception until they have the time and resources to devote to good parenting, so others test their fetus for genetic conditions to avoid a child for whom they don't have the time or money. Such delays, Glover argues, do not express contempt for poor parents or for parents who cannot delay conception. In the same way, couples using assisted reproduction sometimes implant three or four embryos to maximize the chance of any child and sometimes all the embryos take. In the 1997 McCaughey case, where physicians stimulated Mrs. McCaughey's ovaries to superovulate and introduced sperm, they created seven such embryos, which Mrs. McCaughey gestated to become babies. In such a case, many couples agree to selective reduction because they are not prepared to raise seven babies.

Harvard philosopher Frances Kamm distinguishes between loving acceptance of a person who already exists ("caring about" a particular, existing person) and wanting the best qualities in a person yet to exist ("caring to have" the best for a future child).[13] "One can know that one will care about someone just as much whether or not she has certain traits and yet care to have someone, perhaps for their own sake, who has, rather than lacks, those traits." This is because, Kamm says, "Love is for a particular." When we bear a particular child with certain qualities, we love her in all her particularity, and would not substitute another child for her. However, before the existence of a person, there is no one with these particular traits who we must lovingly accept, no one on whom we need to worry about imposing undue expectations.

So the place for high parental expectations is before the child exists. If such expectations are not fulfilled, parents will lovingly accept the existing child in its particularity, because that is the nature of human parental love, which is probably hard-wired into us. No matter what we expect, a newborn baby's face wipes out our previous plans.

In normal life, the door of free will only open a few times. We choose to smoke or, with more difficulty, to give it up; we choose to enter a relationship or, with more difficulty, to end it; we choose a career, or with more difficulty, to change careers. But even these seemingly free choices face many constraints: pressures of time, conditioning, social roles, and limited knowledge. Experts debate how truly free even our most conscious choices are.

This point carries over to choosing traits of future children and love toward existing ones. The door remained shut for most of history about when and whether to have children. Unless one could abstain from sex, children resulted from heterosexual relationships. Only recently did contraception become available, starting with the U. S. Supreme

Court's decision in 1962 in *Griswold vs. Connecticut* that states could not ban physicians from prescribing contraception to married couples and single women. The Roman Catholic Church still attacks that modest advance.[14]

Now the door has been cracked a bit for a few choices about a child's qualities. I say "cracked a bit" because everything points to a very limited ability to predict, much less control, such traits in children, most of which are multi-factorial. But if we can ethically and accurately choose traits, that choice will not take away from the love of existing parents for their particular children.

Alarmists say PGD will bring a Eugenic Armaggedon, but the actual history of PGD shows why we should be skeptical about Alarmist predictions. Why? Because *the scaling problem* matters.

Once we scrutinize questions of scale, PGD does not imply a new Eugenics. The numbers tell the story: IVF is expensive (about $12,000 per attempt) and few states require insurance companies to cover it. Second, it commonly fails: of 100 couples trying IVF, less than 30 will have a baby. Finally, of those thirty couples, it will be the rare couple who will use PGD, and then only if family history or age of mother leads them to suspect a genetic condition.

One of the largest institutes doing PGD over the last decades has only done PGD on 600 couples.[15] Indeed, as several experts testified to the enhancement sessions of the President's Council on Bioethics, scientists *have performed only 6,000 cases in total of PGD between 1990 and 2002.*

Eliminating genetic disease from a few hundred babies a year in America is not going to affect significantly the gene pool of 300 million Americans. Why is that? The numbers are just too large. In 2007, 4,315,000 babies were born in America, up 46,000 from 2006.[16] With so many births passing along so many genes, the small numbers of PGD-related births won't affect the huge genetic mass. In statistical terms, the law of regression to the mean applies. The genes of one baby with a different or missing gene get washed out among the millions of new babies born every year.

Next, whether it's PGD after genetic testing, when a couple chooses against having a child who is blind or deaf for genetic reasons, critics say they "send the wrong message" to people living with these genetic diseases. Is this really so?

Selective perception may be involved here. People choose about thousands of other things that, according to the above logic, also send wrong messages. If couples choose to be childless, does that decision send the message that children are undesirable? If people don't let children in wheelchairs play on soccer teams, does this send the wrong message to children in wheelchairs? Doesn't having a Special Olympics send the wrong message? Doesn't it send the wrong message not to mainstream cognitively challenged children with gifted children? Not to admit people with cognitive disabilities to medical school?

Second, couples make decisions about PGD or abortion *privately.* They don't announce such decisions in the paper. As such, one wonders how such private decisions "send a message" to people with disabilities. If you don't know that I've had a first-term abortion, how can my abortion send a message to you? This is like saying that a person who smokes privately in his own home sends a message that encourages everyone to smoke.

A personal view of the good life may involve raising children, raising children with disabilities, being part of a couple, living alone among others in a city, or being a hermit. Claiming that one of these views of the good life is the *only* good choice confuses morality with personal life, both of which differ from public policy.

Yes, it's a personal decision to have children, but having children is a public good, and the public has a duty to subsidize public education for all children. It also has a right to tax childless couples for such education, and to tax everyone to give special assistance to parents of children with disabilities. Such taxation and subsidy explicitly values children overall and, in particular, children with disabilities, while at the same time reserving liberty to people who choose not to create and raise such children.

Finally, ask yourself this: if there is nothing wrong with spina bifida or cystic fibrosis, should medicine cease trying to cure these conditions? Isn't it contradictory for foundations to appeal for donations for research to cure these conditions, while simultaneously saying there is nothing wrong with the people who have them?

To understand practice X in bioethics, understand the finances surrounding X. Consider who does, or does not, pay for presymptomatic tests for genetic conditions.

Genetic diseases in children cost billions of dollars a year. In a 2004 study, an underlying disorder with a significant genetic component was found in 71 percent of children admitted to a children's hospital for over a year.[17] Any regional children's hospital sees hundreds of children daily who suffer from genetic diseases and who come for surgery, drugs, and therapy. If all such children could have been screened in the womb or as embryos, and healthy embryos/fetuses substituted, and if the same premiums were paid by parents, insurance companies would save billions of dollars a year.

So, financially, and assuming parents may abort, for-profit insurance companies *should* pay for PGD of genetic disease in embryos, genetic testing during the first trimester, and newborn screening. Of course, it's crucial to hold fast to an ethical bright line and not go from *encouraging* parents to test to *requiring* them to test, especially as a condition of keeping coverage.

Paying for genetic tests forces a dilemma on companies that offer medical coverage. Critics will say that genetic testing is only available for the rich. Working people cannot afford to pay $2,000 for a battery of fifty tests to screen out mental retardation. Practically speaking, if medical insurance does not cover such screening, only well-off couples will use it. Economic status is already associated with health, i.e., poverty is associated with disease and early death.[18]

In any effort to prevent genetic disease, physicians will play key roles. In such efforts, they can be seen as the bottleneck, preventing a Eugenic outpouring, or as outdated paternalists who wrongly impose their values on patients.

PGD is not merely a matter of choice of parents; it also involves physicians, adding another layer of complexity. Physicians must deal with malpractice and that matters to such testing.

In the United States, several parents have sued physicians for *wrongful birth*, where lawyers claim some action by physicians made the resulting baby less than normal. Most suits for wrongful birth involve anoxia (lack of oxygen during birth), which may cause cerebral palsy, severe retardation, or vegetative states. Another kind of suit for wrongful birth results from a failure by a physician to inform parents about a test that might have led to a decision not to carry a fetus to term.

At least 27 states allow parents to sue for wrongful birth, although Michigan and Georgia recently disallowed such suits. In 1999, the Georgia Supreme Court ruled that a couple with a child born with Down syndrome or other impairments could not sue their physician for failure to perform amniocentesis or other prenatal tests.[19]

One seminal case concerned Karen Coveler of Houston, Texas, who, at age thirty-four, had earned a doctorate in genetics and who in 2004 requested, "all the DNA tests she could to determine if she was at risk of passing on a genetic disease." [20] Unfortunately, her physician did not offer her a test for her fetus for a genetic cause of deafness, which her son had, leaving him deaf at birth.

Some physicians don't offer similar tests for breast cancer and mental retardation. They make a cost-benefit moral judgment that the genetic condition was not too bad or that the risk of this condition was low, and in their view, the condition did not justify an abortion. Physicians also don't offer such genetic tests in fear that such testing will become the norm—that offering the test will soon become *the standard of care*, such that it is *malpractice* not to offer it. [21]

Consider Fragile X syndrome, a common cause of mental retardation. Unless a family has a history, fetuses are not routinely tested for this condition. Even though Fragile X affects twice as many babies as cystic fibrosis, the American College of Obstetricians and Gynecologists (ACOG) does not, as it does for cystic fibrosis, recommend that most fetuses be tested for it. [22] One critic suggests that ACOG does not do so because, if it did, malpractice claims would fare better against obstetricians who did not test. [23]

Dr. Ronald Librizzi, Chief of Maternal Fetal Medicine at a chain of New Jersey hospitals, regrets that the American College of Obstetricians and Gynecologists recommended that prospective parents test their fetus for cystic fibrosis, but is happy that his hospitals do not offer testing for Fragile X. "I just feel that some people are not ready for some of the information," he said. [24]

All in all, progress in eliminating genetic disease via PGD has been torturously slow, completely unlike the stealth Eugenics predicted by Alarmists. Indeed, one wonders whether such alarmism hasn't made too many parents and physicians overly cautious about testing, resulting in impaired babies that might have been prevented. Sometimes, ethics is part of the problem, not the solution.

To conclude, once again we dissolve Alarmist fears by focusing on one kind of case. Choosing embryos will never create the Master Race because most couples don't use assisted reproduction, it's inefficient and costly, and in three decades, has only been used about 10,000 times in America among 30 million babies born. The effect of any such choices was washed away in the millions of other genes passed along.

NOTES

1. Daniel Kevles, *In the Name of Eugenic: Genetics and the Uses of Human Heredity,* Harvard University Press; Reprint edition (September 1, 1995), 116.ing Man's Estate?" *Journal of the American Medical Association,* 174, no. 19 (November 1971, 779–88.

2. http://www.cdc.gov/mmwr/preview/mmwrhtml/ss5511a1.htm

3. Stephen Mosher, *Broken Earth: The Rural Chinese* (New York: The Free Press, 1984).

4. Hermann Muller, *Out of the Night: A Biologist's View of the Future,* (New York: Vanguard, New York, 1935); quoted in Daniel Kevles, *In the Name of Eugenics,* 164.

5. J. B. S. Haldane, "Toward a Perfected Posterity," *The World Today* 45 (December 1924); quoted in Daniel Kevles, *In the Name of Eugenics,* 122. See also Ronald W. Clark, *The Life and Work of J. B. S. Haldane,* Coward-McCann, New York, 1968, 70.

6. Gunnar Broberg and Nils Roll-Hansen, *Eugenics and the Welfare State: Sterilization Policy in Norway, Sweden, Denmark, and Finland* (Lansing: Michigan State University Press, 1997; revised edition, 2005).

7. Gary Sigley, "'Peasants into Chinamen': Population, Reproduction and Eugenics in Contemporary China." *Asian Studies Review,* no. 3 (1998): 309–38; *Imperfect Conceptions: Medical Knowledge, Birth Defects, and Eugenics in China* (New York: Columbia, 1998); Stephen Garton, "Sound Minds and Healthy Bodies: Re-Considering Eugenics in Australia, 1914–1940," *Australian Historical Studies* 26 (1994): 163–81.

8. Kim Severson, "Payment Set for Those Sterilized in Program," *New York Times,* January 11, 2012, A13.

9. Julie Robotham, "Young Women Seeking Prenatal Tests," *Sydney Morning Herald,* August 30, 2004.

10. Jonathan Glover, *Choosing Children: Genes, Disability, and Design,* (New York: Oxford University Press, 2007).

11. Frances Kamm, "What is and is Not Wrong with Enhancement?" Faculty Research Working Papers Series. John F. Kennedy School of Government, Harvard University, May 2006, RWP06-020, 28.

12. Manya A. Brachear , "Document Clarifies Church's Position on Bioethical Issues," *ChicagoTribune,* December 13, 2008 (also published in *The New York Times* on the same day).

13. Figure is through December, 2003, for the Genetics & IVF Institute of Fairfax, Virginia. See: http://www.givf.com/pgt_sepv.cfm

14. National Center for Health Statistics. http://www.cdc.gov/nchs/pressroom/04facts/pregestimates.htm and http://www.cdc.gov/nchs/data/nvsr/nvsr56/nvsr56_21.htm

15. S. E. McCandless, et al., "The Burden of Genetic Disease on Inpatient Care in a Children's hHspital," *American Journal of Human Genetics* (April 2004), 74, no. 4.

16. Stephen Isaacs and Steven Schroeder "Class—The Ignored Determinant of the Nation's Health," *New England Journal of Medicine,* 351:11, Sept. 9, 2004, 1137–41.

17. "High Court Rules "Wrongful Birth" Suits Invalid," *Atlanta Journal-Constitution,* July 7, 1999, E1.

18. Amy Harmon, "As Gene Test Menu Grows, Who Gets to Choose?" *New York Times,* July 21, 2004, A1, A15.

19. Amy Harmon, "As Gene Test Menu Grows."

20. Also, some data indicate that early diagnosis of cystic fibrosis will lead to decreased morbidity (illness) in people affected, but this is not so with Fragile X syndrome. Also, the genetic test for cystic fibrosis can be done on newborns.

21. Amy Harmon, "As Gene Test Menu Grows," A15.
22. Amy Harmon, "As Gene Test Menu Grows," A15.
23. Amy Harmon, "As Gene Test Menu Grows," A15.
24. Amy Harmon, "As Gene Test Menu Grows," A15.

Chapter Eleven

Eugenic Abortions?

Past Alarmists scandalously predicted that couples would abort normal fetuses to get better, blonde-haired, blue-eyed babies. Such Eugenic abortion would be the terrible, genetic engineering of the human race. For abortion, this is the Nazi objection. In this short chapter, I hope to demonstrate the foolishness of that claim and the myriad reasons why it could never have come true and why it will never come true in the future.

The most important point to stress is exactly the one that Alarmists make, that abortions against genetic conditions such as Tay Sachs, Huntington's disease, Batten's disease, and neural tube defects *are not normal abortions* but done because of what is discovered by prenatal tests on the fetus or fetal fluids. They are "genetic abortions" or "eugenic abortions," where couples choose against Down syndrome, spina bifida, Huntington's disease, perhaps even a deadly neurological condition such as Tay Sachs. Nevertheless, that choice is not alarming.

In these cases, the couples desire a child. They *want* to be pregnant. Unlike 99 percent of abortions, they do not choose *against* pregnancy but against a terrible genetic condition. Their decision is agonizing because they want the child. Their desire for a child conflicts with their appreciation of the difficulty of raising a disadvantaged child.

This is not the same as *choosing for* a specific bundle of traits. That is not possible now. This is negative enhancement, not positive.

Even when they discover an unexpected genetic condition, some couples continue the pregnancy. Why? They may be on their last chance for a child of their own. They may think they can handle the condition. They may decide they just can't abort their fetus.

Despite the claims of Alarmists, most couples make sensible choices after results of these tests: they do not abort because a fetus lacks blonde hair or blue eyes (assuming medicine could test for these traits, which it cannot). In general, the more severe the defect, the greater the reluctance of couples to carry the affected fetus to term. For example, a fetus with neurofibromatosis or Huntington's disease will often be aborted, but not one with Turner syndrome (which can be treated by hormone replacement therapy).

What this shows is how unlikely it is that any kind of stealth Eugenics could be arising from genetic diagnosis in a fetus and followed by abortion. For most cases, the fetus is just too developed, and the couple is just too bonded to it for such decisions to be made on superficial grounds. Indeed, most couples sadly and reluctantly abort only after such a diagnosis.[1]

In 2004, such developments leapt forward, giving couples new options about their future babies. Understanding the significance of these changes requires some background.

The U.S. Supreme Court's 1973 *Roe vs. Wade* analyzed moral value as increasing with age of the fetus; a near-term fetus had much greater value than a two-day-old embryo. This analysis reflects the actual behavior of physicians who perform abortions: many perform early abortions, but not third-trimester abortions. Most would also insert an IUD or prescribe a morning-after pill, but only a tiny few will abort a twenty-week-old fetus.

Until recently, abortions for genetic reasons had to be performed around twenty weeks because that was when amniocentesis results were received. Before twenty weeks, the amniotic sac around the fetus was not big enough to safely insert the needle to withdraw fluid for testing. When results showed a genetic condition such as Down syndrome, couples had to decide at a very late date whether to terminate a planned pregnancy.

Another test, chorionic villus sampling (CVS), takes fetal cells derived from the placenta at about ten weeks of gestation. Because both CVS and amniocentesis cause slightly increased risks of miscarriage (1/100 and 1/300, respectively), some couples avoid both tests.

Amniocentesis, followed by abortion, has been a difficult choice for many couples.[2] Even when they chose abortion, because couples really wanted a baby, the decision traumatized them. For almost six months, the couple's thoughts had been on the expected baby, and the mother had bonded with her fetus. Whatever decision they made, the couple felt guilty.

Beginning in 2004, high-resolution sonograms showed prospective parents remarkable pictures of first-trimester fetuses, and as early as fifteen weeks, some fetuses had human faces and appeared to be smiling. Anti-abortion advocates showed these pictures to dissuade women who contemplated abortions, but the same sonograms also showed neural tube defects such as spina bifida or the characteristic translucent area at the back of the neck of a fetus with Down syndrome.

In the same year, physicians began to use these sonograms with three simple blood tests to determine if a first-trimester fetus had an increased risk of Down syndrome or other genetic condition.[3] This new, multi-stage testing has several important ethical aspects.

First, there is the matter of justification. According to *Roe vs. Wade's* analysis of moral value, the fetus killed in an earlier abortion has less moral value than one killed in the late, second trimester. Second, less weighty reasons are required to justify a first trimester abortion than a late, second-trimester abortion.

This matches what might be called the *gradient view* of personhood. Biologically, we know that the human embryo develops by degrees during the first trimester into a fetus, and then over the next trimester, the fetus grows into viability, and finally, during the last trimester, into a baby. No one event or day along this nine-month journey marks *the* day of personhood. The most accurate view is that personhood accumulates by degrees over time.

On this view, a two-year-old is more of a person than a newborn baby, and a twenty-six-year-old at the height of his powers and health is more of a person than a two-year-old. If personhood depends on capacities, then a human at maximal capacities is more of a person than a human with few capacities.

At the end of life, people lose personhood by degrees, especially with diseases that rob them of their minds. A ninety-year-old man with initial Alzheimer's and an I.Q. of 70 is only "half the man he once was" at age forty-five with an I.Q. of 140. Next, because abortion to avoid genetic disease is one of the best possible reasons for an abortion, such abortions seem more justifiable than normal ones. Altogether, an early genetic abortion seems more justified than a second-trimester abortion of a healthy fetus.

Second, because the abortion is at the end of the first trimester, family, friends, and neighbors need not be aware of the pregnancy. If one family has a history of genetic disease and the couple wishes to consider an abortion, they can keep the pregnancy quiet. Because people fear social condemnation, this privacy matters greatly. If no one knows a wife is pregnant, no third parties can attempt to intervene.

Third, a reasonably priced test now exists for many conditions that cause mental retardation. For more money, Baylor College of Medicine and its associated Quest Genetics can screen fetal cells for more than 450 conditions, including deafness and dwarfism."[4] As said, for Down syndrome, sonograms and blood tests detect 90 percent of cases and, for trisomy 18 (another genetic cause of retardation), 97 percent.[5]

These tests allow couples to test a first-trimester fetus for cystic fibrosis, the most common genetic disease among white couples, and after a positive test, to undergo an early abortion. Other couples abort after learning their child would have Fragile X syndrome.

But every tool works both ways. After high-resolution sonograms were introduced to monitor development of normal pregnancies and to detect genetic abnormalities, groups opposed to abortion realized the potential of the same machines to show powerful images of the young fetus. For example, a "pregnancy counseling center" in Bowie, MD., offered a young, six-and-a-half weeks' pregnant woman inquiring about abortion services a picture of her fetus to check its viability. When the woman heard the fetal heartbeat and saw the images, she decided she could not abort it.[6]

Conservative Christian groups such as James Dobson's Focus on the Family and the Southern Baptist Convention have raised millions of dollars to give such clinics ultrasound machines, which cost about $25,000 each. A group that tracks success of pregnancy centers says that the use of such machines increases their success rate from 70 percent to 90 percent in dissuading women from abortions. About 3,000 such pregnancy-counseling centers, whose primary purpose is not to provide unbiased information regarding all options but rather to dissuade women from having abortions, exist in the United States,.

Some of these pregnancy centers partner with adoption agencies. Adoption agencies cannot explicitly charge for babies—that would be illegal baby-selling—but they can charge substantial sums for arranging the adoption. Standard fees for healthy white babies go as high as $50,000.[7]

■■■

The main point of this chapter is to show why abortion after diagnosis of a genetic defect will never become a Eugenic tidal wave. Abortions are too traumatic and almost all couples choosing genetic abortions wanted a child. Although fetal sonograms may dissuade women from aborting *healthy* fetuses, when combined with other tests, such sonograms convince many parents to abort fetuses with genetic conditions. Again, this is not dangerous. Over the next century, more choice against such conditions may result in much less grief for many families.

NOTES

1. Bill Keller, "Charlie's Ghost," *New York Times*, June 29, 2002.
2. Bill Keller, "Charlie's Ghost," *New York Times*, June 29, 2002.
3. Jane Brody, "Prenatal Tests Now Cheaper, Less Risky," *New York Times*, August 1, 2004.
4. Amy Harmon, "In New Tests for Fetal Defects, Agonizing Choices for Parents," *New York Times Magazine,* June 20, 2004, 2.
5. American College of Obstetricians and Gynecologists Opinion #296, "First Trimester Screening for Fetal Aneuploidy." *Obstetrics and Gynecology* 2004, July, Volume 104, No. 1, 215–17.
6. Neela Banerjee, "Church Groups Turn to Sonogram to Turn Women From Abortion," *New York Times*, February 2, 2005, A1–A5.
7. Neela Banerjee, "Church Groups."

Chapter Twelve

Building Better Kids during Gestation

As explained, too much discussion about enhancement has been sensationalistic talk about babies and choosing genes of embryos. Even to rebut such talk reinforces its bias toward Alarmism.

In the history of medicine, views about the effect of early events in utero on the fetus have swung between two extremes: great vulnerability and relative invincibility. Keating's 1889 *Cyclopedia of the Diseases of Children* gave examples of birth defects due to women being exposed to unpleasant images.[1] For example, the condition of "Elephant Man" Joseph Merrick, was said to have been caused when an elephant frightened his mother at a circus.

By the 1930s, modern medicine had swung to the other extreme, where the pelvic girdle supposedly protected the fetus. Although this pelvic girdle in fact protects the fetus and placenta from physical trauma for the first six months of gestation, after viability the fetus becomes more vulnerable to assault.[2]

In 1941, an Australian physician observed cataracts in babies, a very rare condition, and when he saw several cases, linked it to rubella in their mothers. Greeted with skepticism at first, it took five years for medicine to accept N. McAlester Gregg's hypothesis.

In the early 1960s, women in Europe used thalidomide as a tranquilizer; in the United States, pregnant women used it as an anti-nausea drug. The terrible results taught everyone that drugs cross the placenta and harm babies; in the case of thalidomide, in the form of missing arms and legs. In Arizona in 1962, Sherri Finkbine learned after taking thalidomide that taking it caused babies to be born with missing arms and legs, so she sought a therapeutic abortion. State authorities denied her one, so she went to Sweden to abort a fetus that, in fact, had missing arms and legs.

In 1966, rare cancers started showing up in teenage girls. Soon scientists linked the cancers to diethylstilbestrol (DES), a synthetic estrogen. This drug, widely prescribed for years during pregnancy, did not show its harmful effects until twenty years later, and taught a sobering lesson about the long-term effects of early exposure of the fetus to drugs. Forty-five years later, children and grandchildren still claim that their cancers have been caused by exposure of their mothers and grandmothers to DES.[3]

In some female fetuses with congenital adrenal hyperplasia, the female fetus becomes exposed to testosterone and is virilized as a male.[4] Biologically a woman, this human is later attracted to women as a male and often dresses as a male. This shows the profound influence of early exposure of hormones to the embryo/fetus.

Enhancing humans can be seen from two directions, positive and negative. Consider an analogy with utilitarianism, where moral philosophers distinguish between negative and positive utilitarianism. The former creates the greatest good by eliminating the most suffering, the latter by creating the most happiness. Similarly, we can try to improve humans during gestation either by *negative enhancement*, by removing impediments to fetal flourishing or by *positive enhancement,* by trying to move fetuses to a higher plane.

Enhancing fetuses negatively can be done in two major ways: first, by removing causes of harm during gestation, such as alcohol and smoking, second, by remedying known deficiencies that stunt growth and intelligence, with essential vitamins and minerals such as folic acid and iron.

Let us first consider alcohol. Because of the strength of its lobby, even today we do not fully know the harmful effects of it on children, although even Aristotle knew that its excessive intake harmed babies. For most of the twentieth century, this lobby resisted efforts to prove that drinking by expectant mothers harmed babies.

It took until 1973 for two medical researchers at the University of Washington to prove that alcohol could produce birth defects in babies: smaller heads, lower birth-weight, and a then-new condition called "fetal alcohol syndrome."

In 1977, the National Institute on Alcohol Abuse and Alcoholism issued a report on how alcohol damages fetuses. In 1981, Surgeon General C. Everett Koop flatly declared that women should not drink during pregnancy. In 1989, alcoholic beverages began to contain labels warning women against drinking during pregnancy.

In 1996, the Institute of Medicine (IOM) studied research on women who drank and concluded that more than six drinks a day while pregnant significantly raised the risks of birth defects in newborns. It defined a range of disorders caused by drinking alcohol, calling the whole spectrum "fetal alcohol syndrome" (FAS). The IOM concluded that alcohol may damage the developing fetus the most during the first trimester, when the nervous system and brain developed, resulting in children with poor memory, attention deficit hypersensitivity disorder (ADHD), and mental retardation. In addition, drinking in pregnancy is associated with later problems of teenagers, such as dependence on alcohol and on illegal drugs, poor control of impulses, suicide, and depression.

Over the last fifty years, as knowledge of the damaging effects of alcohol have grown, public campaigns to lower consumption of alcohol in expectant women have lowered the acceptable number of drinks per day from the six drinks in 1977 to two drinks a day to one drink a day to no drinking at all. Today the Centers for Disease Control says,

> When a pregnant woman drinks alcohol, so does her unborn baby. There is no known safe amount of alcohol to drink while pregnant and there also does not appear to be a safe time to drink during pregnancy either. Therefore, it is recommended that women abstain from drinking alcohol at any time during pregnancy.[5]

Unfortunately, women of childbearing age continue to drink, some not knowing they have become pregnant. Binge drinking is consuming more than five drinks a day or an average of forty-five drinks a month. A 2001 survey by the CDC showed that six million women, or 11 percent of women age eighteen to forty-five, binge drank every week. In 2003, that figure rose to 13 percent (7 million women).[6]

As commercials glorify drinking and as more people attend college expecting a holiday before their real life begins, the number of young women who drink heavily rises.

Women who drink heavily fare poorly in negotiating safe sex, and hence, often become pregnant. Such pregnant women sometimes choose to keep their babies. Their subsequent babies are at risk for many developmental disorders. Fetal alcohol syndrome varies among different ethnic groups. One CDC survey reported these rates: Asians 0.3, Hispanics 0.8, whites 0.9, blacks 6.0, and Native Americans 29.9.[7] This rate in Native Americans—nearly 30 per 10,000 births—should not be interpreted to mean that the rate is the same for all tribes: "Reports from health units that serve Navajo and Pueblo tribes indicate a prevalence of FAS that is similar to that of the general population in the U.S., but the prevalence reported among the Southwest Plains Indians was much higher (1 per 102 live births)."

There is also evidence that men who drink heavily while trying to conceive can affect their future fetus through their abnormal sperm.[8] It is even also possible that the genes of such heavy drinkers may affect their grandchildren.[9]

This is a touchy subject, as people realize they drank while they conceived or gestated their children. Until recently, the dangers of alcohol during conception and pregnancy were not appreciated.

Now consider smoking. Besides alcohol, removing nicotine from fetuses would be a negative fetal enhancement. Incidence of cleft palate can be graphed according to how many packs of cigarettes a pregnant woman smokes.[10] Maternal smoking during pregnancy is associated later with Type 2 diabetes, obesity, and mental retardation.[11] Even secondhand smoke harms the fetus.[12]

Now let us consider correcting deficiencies of nutrition in utero. In July 2008, a remarkable article appeared in the *New England Journal of Medicine*, "Effect of In Utero and Early-Life Conditions on Adult Health and Disease."[13] Medicine has long known that environmental triggers can activate genetic predispositions to disease, even decades after birth. These authors argued that such triggers started osteoporosis, cardiovascular disease, and metabolic diseases such as diabetes.

They concluded that "environmental factors acting during [early] development should be accorded greater weight in models of disease causation." Their meta-study of hundreds of animal and human studies showed that solid medical evidence exists that many common chronic diseases can be prevented by making surprisingly simple changes during gestation and the first years of a baby's life.

Vitamins came to be in food today by a long path. They are definitely good for human fetuses and babies. Around 1870, some scientists started to believe that the body could not thrive only on carbohydrates, fats, proteins, and mineral salts. They hypothesized that the body's health required some other mysterious, vital substance. Whatever these mysterious substances were, lack of them seemed to cause serious diseases. Then in 1906, Axel Holst, a bacteriologist in Oslo, and Frederick Hopkins in England, hypothesized that lack of such vital substances caused diseases such as beriberi, scurvy, pellagra, and ricketts. [14]

In 1912, Caismir Funk of London's Lister Institute called these (in the mistaken belief that they derived from ammonia) "vital amines." When scientists later realized that not all vitamins were amines, they dropped the "e."

Jumping forward almost a century to 1995, scientists then discovered that taking folic acid during pregnancy reduced the number of babies born with neural tube defects. [15] As explained in the preface, Canada, whose eastern provinces had historically suffered high rates of such neural tube defects, mandated in 1998 the fortification of wheats and cereals with folic acid. Later studies showed that this was wise. Such fortification decreased the incidence of neural tube defects by almost half, with the greatest number decrease in the eastern provinces. [16]

The Institute of Medicine recommended in 1998 that expectant women every day consume 600 micrograms of folic acid. [17] Many prenatal vitamins today contain up to 1,000 micrograms of folic acid. [18]

Wouldn't it be nice if scientists had simply discovered that folic acid reduces impaired babies, government had acted on this discovery, and the public health had been quickly improved? In fact, as FDA historian Susan White Junod documents, makers of natural foods and supplements battled for years against professional nutritionists, pediatricians, and scientists. [19] Part of the issue involved medicating the entire population and proving no harm from doing so. Another part involved proving benefit to babies, proving the correct dosage, and proving what methods of delivery worked best.

Given the claims now about such mass introductions of vitamins, vaccinations, fluoridation of water, and exposure to substances such as mercury, it is easy to see why a national program in the 1990s to eradicate a disease caused by a nutritional deficiency raised ethical alarms. For any such substance introduced in food, water, or by vaccination, a few people will experience adverse reactions, even anaphylactic shock and death. Authorities in public health must extensively justify their utilitarian judgment that prevention of the harm to the huge majority justifies risk of inflicting harms on the unlucky few.

But let's return to our story of folic acid. By 1991, some physicians knew that folic acid reduced spina bifida and anencephaly, the two most common neural tube defects in babies, by 50 to 70 percent. A randomized, multinational trial run by Britain's Medical Research Council had that year published such results in the *Lancet*.[20] Based on that study and other evidence, the Centers for Disease Control recommended in 1991 that pregnant women take four milligrams of folic acid each day to prevent neural tube defects.

The problem concerned how to get the folic acid to them, especially as evidence mounted that to work its purpose, a woman needed to take folic acid before she got pregnant or immediately thereafter. Since many pregnancies were unplanned, this posed a problem. Also, as babies with neural tube defects occurred more commonly among poor women, this made impractical programs where at-risk women took folic acid by prescription or by expensive supplements.

Since World War II, the U.S. government and the Food and Drug Administration (FDA) had required several additions to the public's food to prevent disease and defects in babies. As historian Suzanne Junod writes, these included:

> Iodine ... added to salt in 1924 to prevent goiter. In the 1930s, vitamin D ... to milk to prevent ricketts and [to] aid in calcium and phosphorus absorption. From 1938 through 1943, an enrichment formula was developed for flours and breads that included thiamin to prevent berberi, niacin to prevent pellagra, riboflavin to assist in B6 and niacin utilization, and iron to prevent anemia. Later, vitamin D was added to low and non-fat diary products and lysine has been added to a few foods to enhance their protein content, but such additions ...[were] few and far between in the aftermath of the impressive World War II initiatives.[21]

In many ways, the public's naïve trust in government and medicine during World War II helped enhance the health of its babies. Giving present skepticism about governmental programs, introducing new fetal enhancements today presents more difficulties.

We still must climb a big hill. Even today, most pregnant women in the United States, let alone the rest of the world, don't take folic acid. In 2005, only 33 percent of childbearing-aged women took it during their pregnancies, down from 40 percent in 2004.[22] Among women eighteen to twenty-four years of age, over 60 percent knew nothing about folic acid, and only 6 percent knew when it's best to take it.[23] In Puerto Rico, where the prevalence of neural tube defects in babies exceeds that of the United States, and despite campaigns to change the problem, only one fourth of pregnant women take folic acid.[24] Clearly, we have a long way to go for just one simple enhancement.

In 2010, a remarkable study by Christopher Eppig investigated the burden of disease around the world on developing intelligence in children.[25] First they mapped out the lowest average intelligence scores and found them to be in Equatorial Guinea, St. Lucia, Cameroon, Mozambique, and Gabon. The highest were in Japan, South Korea, Singapore, China, Europe, and the United States.

What they discovered was a correlation between average intelligence and the burden of disease. The correlation, which is not direct causation, was very high, 67 percent. It is higher than contributions of income, education of parents, climate, agricultural labor, and distance from mankind's origins.

The authors hypothesize that the development of a child's brain requires 87 percent of its body's metabolic energy. Any sickness during gestation or at birth, or in the early years of its brain's development, hijacks its ability to develop.

We already know that intestinal worms and malaria suffered during infancy harm human brains. Surprisingly, diseases that cause diarrhea may harm the developing brain the most, depriving it of essential nutrients at key times.

The implications of Eppig's research are that a country's intelligence can be raised by curing its infectious diseases. Bismarck was right: an efficient public health system, backed by public hospitals, is the backbone of a nation's long-term strength. Infectious diseases kill its children and stunt survivors with retardation.

It is a shame that more evidence has not been gathered. Obviously, ethics blocks some research. For example, you cannot do a prospective, randomized clinical trial, where half the mothers are urged not to breastfeed, as their children might be damaged. Nevertheless, it is disappointing that, in this age of huge research budgets and many foundations, more evidence is not being gathered for an issue that might deeply affect the 135 million humans born each year and their families.[26]

If we really want to get serious about enhancing all humans, not just North Americans, we will rapidly get the world's food fortified in certain basic ways. A great advance in the world's intelligence could be achieved simply by assuring that every pregnant mother and baby gets enough iodine, especially through using iodized salt. Hundreds of millions of people in India and Asia lack diets with enough iodine, and even a small deficiency of iodine can lower a child's IQ by 10 to 15 points.[27] Lack of iodine is the world's leading preventable cause of mental retardation. Later, when the damage manifests itself in childhood, it cannot be reversed.

Even more dramatically, lack of iron may affect as many as two billion people worldwide. Supplementing wheat flour with iron could prevent iron deficiency, the most common nutritional deficiency on the planet and one that prevents formation in the body of sufficient hemoglobin. Lack of iron may delay or impede development in children and may cause anemia in adults that can damage organs.

Because humans around the world consume more wheat flour than any other cereal grain, fortification of such flour with folic acid, iron, and essential vitamins is a simple enhancement that can prevent a vast amount of retardation and disease at an amazingly low cost.[28] Despite continuing efforts by various agencies to increase access of humans to such fortified flour, and some success (a half a billion more people ate such flour in 2007 than in 2004), nearly two-thirds of the world's population still lacks access to fortified wheat flour.

Finally, steps can be taken in utero to try to positively enhance fetuses. For example, during the last trimester of pregnancy and the first months after birth, the fetal brain undergoes a spurt of growth and increases its content of the fatty acids docosahexaenoic acid (DHA) and arachidonic acid (AA). Some studies suggest that if the mother's diet is poor in these fatty acids, children may be born with low IQs. Conversely, supplementing the maternal diet during pregnancy with such fatty acids may increase a child's intelligence.

In a study published in 2003 in *Pediatrics*, mothers taking fish oil DHA and AA during pregnancy had children who at age four scored four points higher on IQ tests than children of similar mothers who only took corn oil during pregnancy. A 2007 *Lancet* study followed nearly 12,000 British women and discovered that those who ate three portions of fish per week during pregnancy produced children with higher IQs and who developed better than the children of other pregnant women who ate no seafood.

Another review of eight randomized clinical trials in 2007 revealed that expectant mothers who took fish oil during pregnancy increased the IQ of their children up to four points. Unfortunately, a meta-study in 2011 found no long-term, beneficial effects on IQ from fish oil.[29] As of 2012, the effect of taking fish oil during pregnancy on children's IQ remains unresolved.

There is a great deal more to know about fetal enhancement. Some of the most obvious measures that might increase a child's lifelong prospects have not been scientifically proven. In a review in 2002 in *Pediatrics* of forty studies between 1929 and 2001 of the effect of breast-feeding on a child's intelligence, the authors used eight principles of epidemiology to evaluate if any real evidence could be found.[30] Unfortunately, only two studies were judged capable of producing reliable data, and of these, one inferred a significant effect of breast-feeding on intellect, but the other did not.

The main idea advanced by this chapter has been that, to improve future humans, we need not experiment with risky genetic interventions because a great deal can be done now to remove what harms both fetuses and newborn children. Simply by adding folic acid, iron, and iodine to meals, we could prevent many kinds of birth defects. By getting pregnant women to abstain from smoking and drinking during pregnancy, we could raise IQs and prevent many adult-onset diseases. Finally, if we could get the minimal amount of iodine, nutrition, and food to the world's pregnant women, who knows how healthy and bright we might make the average human child?

NOTES

1. John M. Keating (ed), *Cyclopedia of the Diseases of Children: Medical and Surgical.* 1889 (Philadelphia, Pa: Lippincott, 1889), vol. III.
2. My points here are indebted to conversations with UAB professor of Obstetrics and Gynecology Kim Hoover and also the Ann McMillan Lecture at UAB by NIH epidemiologist Allen Wilcox on March 2, 2011, in the Hill University Center.
3. Sarah Morrison and Jaymi McCann, "Thousands of Women Could Be at Risk from 'Silent Thalidomide'," *The Independent* (London, England), January 22, 2012.
4. A big controversy in bioethics surrounds this issue. See the Web site for fetaldex at: http://fetaldex.org/home.html
5. Centers for Disease Control, "Fetal Alcohol Spectrum Disorders," http://www.cdc.gov/ncbddd/fas/default.htm
6. J. Tsai , R.L. Floyd, & J. Bertrand. "Tracking Binge Drinking among U.S. Childbearing-age Women." *Preventive Medicine* (April 2007), 44, no. 4, 298–302.

7. G. F. Chavez, J. F. Cordero, & J. E. Becerra, "Leading major congenital malformations among minority groups in the United States, 1981–1986," *Journal of the American Medical Association* (1989) 261, no. 2, 205–09.

8. Katy Sinclair, "Sperm Damage Can be Passed to Children," *BioNews-IVF News,* February 26, 2008.

9. John Cloud, "Why Your DNA Isn't Your Destiny," *Time,* January 6, 2010.

10. "Smoking and Orofacial Clefts: A United Kingdom–Based Case-Control Study," 10.1597/02-142. *The Cleft Palate-Craniofacial Journal:* 41:4, 381–86.

11. Scott Montgomery, "Smoking During Pregnancy and Diabetes Mellitus in a British Longitudinal Birth Cohort," *British Medical Journal* 324, January 5, 2002, 26–27.

12. WebMD Health News, "Secondhand Smoke May Harm Fetus Like Smoking, Study Shows Passive Smoking Just as Risky as Smoking by Pregnant Women," July 27, 2005.

13. P. Gluckman et al., "Effect of In Utero and Early-Life Conditions on Adult Health and Disease." *New England Journal of Medicine,* 359, no. 1, July 3, 2008, 62–73.

14. Roy Porter, *The Greatest Benefit to Mankind: A Medical History of Humanity* (New York: Norton, 1997), 554.

15. G.M. Shaw et al, "Periconceptional Vitamin Use, Dietary Folate, and the Occurrence of Neural Tube Defects," *EPGDemiology* (1995). 6, no. 3, 219–22.

16. Philippe De Wals, "Reduction in Neural Tube Defects after Folic Acid Fortification in Canada," *New England Journal of Medicine* 357, July 12, 2007, 135–42.

17. M. A. Paulozzi et al., Impact of Folic Acid Fortification on the US Food Supply on the Occurrence of Neural Tube Defects," *Journal of the American Medical Association* (2001), 285, 2981-986.

18. Institute of Medicine. Food and Nutrition Board. *Dietary Reference Intakes: Thiamin, Riboflavin, Niacin, Vitamin B6, Folate, Vitamin B12, Pantothenic Acid, Biotin, and Choline.* (Washington, D.C.: National Academy Press. 1998).

19. Susan White Junod, "Folic Acid Fortification: Fact and Folly," Update, the bimonthly publication of the Food and Drug Law Institute. http://www.fda.gov/oc/history/makinghistory/folicacid.html

20. Medical Research Council. "Folic Acid Study," *Lancet,* 1991.

21. Susan White Junod, "Folic Acid Fortification," p. 5 (print version of online article).

22. Centers for Disease Control, "Use of Dietary Supplements Containing Folic Acid Among Women of Childbearing Age—United States, 2005," *Morbidity and Mortality Report,* (September 30, 2005), 54, no. 38, 955–958.

23. Centers for Disease Control, "Use of Supplements Containing Folic Acid Among Women of Childbearing Age—United States, 2007," *Morbidity and Mortality Report,* January 11, 2008 57, no. 1, 5–8.

24. Centers for Disease Control, "Prevalence of Neural Tube Defects and Folic Acid Knowledge and Consumption—Puerto Rico, 1996-2006, *Morbidity and Mortality Report,* January 11, 2008 57, no. 1, 10–13.

25. "Mens Sana in Corpore Sano," *The Economist,* July 3, 2010, 75.

26. U. S. Census Bureau, "World Vital Events: World Vital Events Per Time Unit: 2008." http://www.census.gov/cgi-bin/ipc/pcwe

27. Donald G. McNeil, Jr. "Raising the World's IQ: The Secret's in the Salt," *New York Times,* December 15, 2006.

28. Centers for Disease Control, "Trends in Wheat-Flour Fortification with Folic Acid and Iron—Worldwide, 2004 and 2007, *Morbidity and Mortality Report* (January 11, 2008), 57, no. 1, 8–10.

29. Maria Makrides et al., "Effect of DHA Supplementation During Pregnancy on Maternal Depression and Neurodevelopment of Young Children: A Randomized Controlled Trial, *Journal of the American Medical Association* (2010), 304, no. 15, 1675–683.

30. Anjali Jain et al, "How Good is the Evidence Linking Breastfeeding and Intelligence?" *Pediatrics* 109, no. 6, June 2002, 1044–54.

Chapter Thirteen

Building Better Kids: Vaccinations

Let's now briefly consider vaccinations at birth to improve humans. Exposure to a tiny amount of a disease causes the immune system to build a response and to remember that exposure. Such vaccination permanently changes a person's cells. No wonder people initially feared it; it is irrevocable.

Vaccinations do not cure a disease in a specific patient; rather, they prevent a disease in possible patients. As such, vaccinations prove that we can intervene in humans, even children and babies, not just to cure disease but to prevent its start.

Vaccinations enhance, in the negative sense, by preventing something bad and hence, indirectly elevating normal health.

The justification of mass vaccination against infectious diseases depends on utilitarianism, the belief that morally correct actions produce the greatest good for the greatest number of people. The justification also depends on knowledge of medical history.

The best way to appreciate mundane vaccines is to focus on what happened in 1918 when no flu vaccine existed. In one month, influenza killed 400,000 Americans, most under the age of thirty. [1] By the time it had swept the planet, it had killed 50 to 200 million people—between 3 and 6 percent of the world's population. About 500 million more suffered from it and thought they might die. [2] In India alone, 20 million children died.

In the last century, two of the great, little-known heroes were agricultural scientist Norman Borlaug and vaccine-developer Maurice Hilleman. Norman Borlaug developed a form of dwarf wheat in the 1960s that could grow plentifully in bad conditions, sparking the Green Revolution and preventing a then-predicted global starvation that might have killed a billion people.[3] Thanks to biotechnology, food-importing countries such as India, China, and the Philippines became self-sufficient.

As virologist Paul Offit details in *Vaccinated*, Maurice Hilleman is the other unsung hero of the last half of the twentieth century.[4] Before he began his work in the late 1950s, millions of children and adults worldwide were struck down by measles, mumps, rubella (German measles), chickenpox, hepatitis A and B, pneumococcus, meningococcus, and type b influenza. These diseases killed, paralyzed, deafened, or injured for life. Because of Hilleman's work, we know how to quickly create a safe vaccine against the deadly flu that killed so many in 1918. As the movie *Contagion* showed in 2011, whether a flu epidemic like it occurs again will depend on whether we have the will to combat it early.

Consider the world at the time of the American Revolution, before Edward Jenner created the first vaccine against smallpox. At that time, deadly infectious diseases, such as smallpox, yellow fever, diptheria, tetanus, whooping cough, and polio killed millions worldwide. Because they had no prior immunity, the Native American population dropped from 10 million to 400,000 between 1600 and 1900. What killed them? Yellow fever, measles, smallpox, cholera, and other imported diseases,

Edward Jenner developed the first smallpox vaccine in the late 1700s. Received controversially, its success in saving lives gradually won it adherents, as seen in the HBO series, *John Adams*.[5] It is important to note that the smallpox vaccination is a *biological* enhancement that people now trust.

A century later, Louis Pasteur created the world's second vaccine, this time against rabies. Between 1900 and 1957, scientists created bacterial vaccines against diptheria, tetanus, and some strains of whooping cough. At the end of World War II, they created the first vaccine against flu; in the 1950s, Jonas Salk and Albert Sabin created a vaccine against poliomyelitis.

The most recently developed vaccine was created to combat human papillomavirus (HPV), known to cause cervical cancer. This vaccine created controversy because of its cost (about $140) and because it had to be given to young girls before onset of sexual activity. Vaccines against malaria and the various strains of HIV remain to be created.

Around 1900, public officials recognized the need for mass vaccinations to prevent epidemics among those living in crowded, unsanitary places. Public health officers, sometimes backed by policemen, vaccinated the poor and their children involuntarily in slums, migrant camps, and schools. This created an anti-vaccination fire that has never burned out, in some cases combining assertions of individual bodily rights with religious freedom and fear of medicine, especially by minorities.[6]

Maurice Hilleman entered the world's history again when the Asian flu broke out in southwestern China in February 1957. As it spread eastward to the Philippines and onto U. S. Navy ships, Hilleman knew that only a vaccine would check its spread and, on May 22, appealed to start one.[7] He convinced drug companies to make a vaccine, and by July, 40 million dosages were ready. That fall, 20 million Americans contracted the Asian flu, but thanks to Hilleman's work, only 70,000 died.

Over the next thirty years, Hilleman created two dozen vaccines for infectious diseases, beginning with mumps. Since 1967, when Hilleman's vaccine for mumps began to be used, "more than one hundred fifty million dosages have been distributed in the United States. By 2000, his mumps vaccine had prevented a million children from getting mumps every year, thus every year preventing meningitis and deafness in thousands."[8]

But the history of vaccinations is not one that Enthusiasts can champion without qualification. Hilleman tested his vaccine in the same way that hepatitis vaccines would later be tested: on children in institutions for the cognitively challenged. Indeed, between 1930 and 1970, scientists often tested their vaccines on mentally impaired children.

Today, we would consider such children paradigms of vulnerable populations because they are captive, unable to consent, and dependent on the state or charity for custodial care. On grounds of justice, critics think it wrong that such children be used as guinea pigs for vaccines that, if successful, would benefit the majority of children.

On the other hand, because of their confinement, any infectious disease quickly spreads among such children. Because of difficulties in maintaining hygiene, it is impossible to protect uninfected children from contact with infected children. Because of cognitive impairment, normal attempts to control the spread of infection often are useless. For these reasons, Hilleman felt justified in using these children. Moreover, his intention was therapeutic. In addition, because he was successful, the children benefitted. Saul Krugman argued the same about his hepatitis B vaccination of similar children at the Willowbrook facility on Staten Island, New York, one of the classic cases in bioethics.[9]

Use of captive populations to test vaccines always has its risks, and in the 1940s, the first vaccine against yellow fever suffered contamination with hepatitis B. American servicemen during World War II had no choice but to get this vaccination, and as a result, 300,000 got hepatitis B, of whom at least 60 died as a direct result.[10] The contamination occurred because human serum had been used to stabilize the vaccine against yellow fever. Afterward and because of these deaths, human serum was never used again.

Perhaps the most infamous accidental infection occurred with Jonas Salk's polio vaccine. His vaccine was essentially a very weakened version of the polio virus, which conferred later immunity. But in making the vaccine, one manufacturer, Cutter, failed to properly kill the live virus and inadvertently created a batch of vaccine with a live polio virus that infected 100,000 children, who in turn spread the infectious disease to other children, resulting in another 100,000 infected. In the end, the Cutter-vaccine-with-live-virus killed 10 children, permanently paralyzed 200, and sickened 70,000. Pictures of children forced to live in iron lungs—the first artificial ventilators—scared people and stiffened resistance to mandatory vaccination.

As said, utilitarianism justifies mass vaccinations. Consider measles, which in 1965 killed 8 million children worldwide. Even if a vaccine killed 1 percent of children vaccinated, it would be justified on utilitarian grounds. If it only killed 0.1 percent, the justification deepens. If, when problems were being found, it only killed 0.1 percent in the initial phase, its justification looks very solid. Finally, if a pure vaccine could be created which rarely killed any child, vaccination of all children worldwide would be mandatory.

That is essentially what has happened, and today measles vaccine prevents 7 to 8 million deaths in childhood every year. But there were bumps along this road. Measles vaccine had to be grown in eggs of chickens, and such eggs could be easily contaminated. In one case, the first vaccine became contaminated by a chicken leukemia virus, similar to the one in cats. The key to success was a drug company's purchase of a large, contamination-free chicken farm and use of its eggs to produce the vaccine. Today the Moraten strain still comes from chickens whose ancestors lived at Kimberly Farms.

Hilleman went on to create vaccines against rubella, which between 1963 and 1964 infected 12 million Americans. In this case and as in rabies, chickenpox, and hepatitis A, researchers developing new vaccines used tissue from aborted human fetuses. Such usage angered the Catholic Church and some U.S. evangelicals.

German measles at the time would have been expected to harm 80 percent of the fetuses of the hundreds of thousands of pregnant women it infected, causing miscarriage, retardation, blindness, epilepsy, and autism. A fetus infected with German measles would have been a primary candidate for a genetic abortion.

Fortunately, the rubella vaccine worked well and prevented many deaths, in part because no animal viruses contaminated it. Stanley Plotkin, the virologist who created it by using aborted human fetuses, unapologetically defended its creation against critics: "Frankly, I think that our rubella vaccine has prevented more abortions than all the anti-abortionists put together."[11]

We now assume eradication of formerly lethal, infectious diseases. That diptheria or measles could suddenly kill a million American children is inconceivable. Mass vaccinations have proven remarkably safe and saved millions of lives. They prevented untold suffering.

Unfortunately, vaccination is under attack today. First, for reasons outlined above, some people fear that any vaccine will be contaminated and the vaccine will be worse than the disease.

Second, because of a remarkable case of medical fraud, one in five U.S. and U.K. parents believe that contaminants in vaccines cause autism.[12] In 1998, a paper by English physician Andrew Wakefield argued that a vaccine against measles-mumps-rubella caused autism and other disorders. In the judgment of the editors who published his original article, Wakefield not only committed "bad science," but also "deliberate fraud." His views were undoubtedly influenced by money given to him by a lawyer involved in suing the manufacturer of the vaccine. In 2010, Wakefield was barred from practicing medicine in the United Kingdom.

Today, the weight of medical evidence stands strongly against Wakefield. He is no misunderstood Ignaz Semmelweis or Stanley Prusiner; rather, he is a fraud. He resembles the South African physician who made up data showing that bone marrow transplants could cure recalcitrant breast cancer, thereby causing thousands of women with breast cancer to needlessly undergo such transplants.[13] Because it scares parents about all childhood vaccinations, Wakefield's fraudulent claim will harm children who later get sick because of lack of vaccination.

People who don't vaccinate their children actually depend on most children getting vaccinated to shield their child from exposure; their children benefit from *herd immunity*. Because each and every child does not need to be vaccinated to protect a population from infection, sometimes only 95 or 99 percent is enough (although to eliminate a disease such as polio permanently from the world, *all* children must be vaccinated, or a reservoir of infection will continue).

But if enough parents don't vaccinate, herd immunity decreases, mutations rise, and soon measles, whooping cough, or diphtheria will kill again. In 2010, the CDC reported that *40 percent* of U.S. parents of young children had refused or delayed one or more vaccines for their child.[14] This is one area of enhancement where the United States is moving backward. It is also one area, as *Contagion* illustrated, where the Internet does more harm than good, because anyone can claim anything and others will believe him.

Interestingly, parents who resist vaccinations because they believe that something in vaccines causes autism spectrum disorders may also resist taking folic acid during pregnancy. However, a new, look-back study in late 2011 showed that, in mothers and children with genetic variants that affect how folic acid is metabolized, not taking prenatal folic acid before conception increased the risk of a child with autism by *seven times*.[15]

Historically, mass vaccinations against infectious diseases saved millions of lives of children and prevented millions more from being sick and disabled. Although ethical lapses occurred in development of past vaccines, we are now able to quickly produce safe vaccines that have few downsides.

We now have two vaccines against cancer, one of which is controversial (the one preventing HPV and later, cervical cancer). If we develop a dozen more, will we have the guts to protect future citizens with them?

NOTES

1. K.D. Patterson and G. F. Pyle "The Geography and Mortality of the 1918 Influenza Pandemic" *Bull Hist Med.* (Spring 1991) 65 (1): 4–21.

2. Jeffery K. Taubenberger and David M. Morens, Centers for Disease Control and Prevention, *1918 Influenza: The Mother of All Pandemics*, January 2006. Retrieved on May 9, 2009. Archived 2009-10-01.

3. Gregory Pence and Joyce Hsu, "A Hero for Our Time," *Birmingham News*, July 23, 2000.

4. Paul Offit, *Vaccinated: One Man's Quest to Defeat the World's Deadliest Diseases*, (New York: Smithsonian/Collins Books, 2997).

5. David McCullough, *John Adams* (New York: Simon & Schuster, 2001).

6. Maurice Willrich, *Pox: An American History*, Penguin, 2011, New York.

7. Paul Offit, *Vaccinated: One Man's Quest to Defeat the World's Deadliest Diseases*, 2007, Smithsonian/Collins Books, New York, 14–15.

8. Paul Offit, *Vaccinated*, 30.

9. Saul Krugman, "The Willowbrook hepatitis studies revisited: Ethical aspects," *Reviews of Infectious Diseases* (Jan-Feb, 1986), 8, no. 1:157–62.

10. Paul Offit, *Vaccinated*, 40.

11. Paul Offit, *Vaccinated*, 91.

12. Michael Willrich, "Why Parents Fear the Needle," *New York Times*, January 21, 2011, A23.

13. Richard Rettig et al., *False Hope: Bone Marrow Transplantation for Breast Cancer* (New York: Oxford University Press, 2007.

14. Daniel J. DeNoon,, "More Parents Refuse, Delay Childhood Vaccinations," May 55, 2010, *WebMD Health News.*

15. Rebecca J. Schmidt et. al., "Prenatal Vitamins, One-carbon Metabolism Gene Variants, and Risk for Autism," *Epidemiology*, July 2011, 22, no. 4, 476–85.

Chapter Fourteen

Building Better Emerging Minds: Adderall and Ritalin

Let us now turn to boosting the mental capacity of pre-adults: children, adolescents, and college students. These young people characteristically compete for prizes, degrees, and honors, but how far can we *ethically* maximize their mental enhancement?

Let's note that we already enhance the minds of children in many ways: by talking to babies during infancy, by sending children to preschool classes and enrichment programs, by selecting good schools, by getting both parents and grandparents involved in upbringing, by hiring tutors and special instructors, by finding mentors, and in many other ways. All these efforts aim at producing smarter, more accomplished children.

In the history of discussions of this issue, we see the familiar mistake of lumping together different kinds of enhancement. In 2007, the British Medical Association issued a paper on ethical aspects of cognitive enhancements.[1] It mentioned that such enhancements may have side effects that harm young, developing brains, but a few sentences later, mentioned that germ-line genetic interventions may wrongly alter future humans. This is like talking about giving kids Ritalin in the same paragraph as performing cosmetic brain surgery on them. Different orders of risk should carry different orders of concern.

Millions of children and young adults now take attention-focusing drugs. Critics see such usage as an unjustified mass experiment on vulnerable beings. We certainly need to understand what is happening before recommending even more drugs for such children.

Usage of such drugs in children and in young adults raises new issues because they can't resist pressure as easily as adults, may desire intensely to excel, and may be forced to live with decisions made for them by adults.

The American Psychiatric Association (APA) estimates that Attention Deficit Hypersensitivity Disorder (ADHD) affects approximately 3 to 5 percent of school-age children, 75 percent of whom are boys. It believes that ADHD follows 50 to 80 percent of kids into adolescence and 30 to 50 percent into adult years.[2] Such kids need to be maintained either on Ritalin or Adderall, which allow them to function well in college. This pattern explains why Ritalin and Adderall are the easiest drugs to obtain on campus for nontherapeutic uses.

Patented in 1954 by CIBA pharmaceuticals, methylphenidate, or its better-known trademarked name, Ritalin, began to be used by child psychiatrists during the 1960s to treat children with ADHD. Methylphenidate often improved both mental concentration and calmed mood. Without the drug, lack of focus seemed to cause both poor concentration and hyper-distraction in ADHD kids. By 1998, Ritalin had been prescribed for 5 million American children.[3] In tracking both adult and child prescriptions for methylphenidate and dextroamphetamine for thirty-six months between 2003 and 2006, the FDA discovered that U.S. doctors wrote 80 million prescriptions.[4]

Besides Ritalin, the second most-prescribed cognitive enhancer in children is Adderall, composed of dextroamphetamine, whose active ingredient is an amphetamine salt. Adderall was originally marketed to Americans as the weight-control drug Obetrol. In 1996, Obetrol was marketed for children with ADHD as Adderall.

Both dextroamphetamine and methylphenidate act on the brain in ways like methamphetamine by releasing large quantities of dopamine.[5] Scientists do not agree about exactly how Ritalin works, but it seems to increase the brain's transmission of dopamine. When something exciting happens, such as winning big on a slot machine, the brain releases dopamine and we feel ecstatic.

Methylphenidate is a controversial drug. Some parents claim that using it killed their children.[6] Over the last decade, dozens of stories have exposed ties between pharmaceutical companies and research psychiatrists, leading critics to suspect many studies of the efficacy and safety of Ritalin and Adderall.

Enthusiasts claim Ritalin and Adderall are universal enhancers that could benefit everyone. Methylphenidate seems to allow adults and children to focus; hence, it gives them control over bad impulses. Transhumanist and bioethicist James Hughes claims that both he and his son, by starting to take Ritalin as children, learned to read, to focus, and to be productive (and presumably, they still take it to do so).[7]

Some researchers think that more accurate diagnoses finally revealed the true incidence of ADHD in the United States and thus more children were prescribed Ritalin. The expansion of state Children's Health Insurance Programs (S-CHIP) also explains this increase, as more and more poor children became covered for seeing psychiatrists and getting low-cost prescriptions.

Pediatrician Laurence Diller, a long-time critic and author of *Running on Ritalin: A Physician Reflects on Children, Society and Performance in a Pill,* argues that too many children receive a diagnosis of ADHD and are then put on Ritalin.[8] Rather than getting Ritalin, Diller advocates using love and discipline by two parents, a far more time-consuming and emotionally exhausting approach. He also advocates using behavioral approaches first, especially for pre-school children.[9]

Of course, it's easy to take cheap shots at parents and psychiatrists who put children on Ritalin or Adderall. If both parents need to work to put food on the table and pay the mortgage, and if the alternative to these drugs is that the child can no longer attend public school, the drugs seem like a blessing.

Here's the essential question: are these children the victims of one of the most massive experiments in the history of medicine or are they the beneficiaries of cognitive enhancers that everyone could use? Critics say that enhancing drugs should go to the needy first. Have we done just that with millions of children with ADHD?

Consider this surprising side-fact: right now in medical school, psychiatrists diagnose 2 to 3 percent of medical students with ADHD. Before admission and through effort, these intelligent people could overcome ADHD, but medical school slams them with huge amounts of memorization. When they turn to psychologists for help, they realize they have ADHD. When they get methylphenidate or modafinil, as well as extra time for tests, they perform satisfactorily.

In one of the most critical and extensive investigations of the use of methylphenidate and dextroamphetamine in children, veteran reporter Judith Warner accepted Diller's criticisms above and spent five years writing a book trying to back them up. What she discovered surprised her, and she completely reversed her initial position. As she says in the preface to her 2010 *We've Got Issues: Children and Parents in the Age of Medication:*

> When I first began this book in February 2004, I bought into that story. I was one of the many people who regarded ADHD, bipolar disorder, and the milder variants of the autistic spectrum as "fashionable maladies" of questionable reality. I would, perhaps, not have been quite as blunt as Rush Limbaugh, when he described ADHD as "the perfect way to explain the inattention, incompetence, and inability of adults to control their kids," but my opinions weren't all that far off from his views.
>
> I am embarrassed to admit to that commonality of belief today. I cringe, thinking back on the company that I was prepared to keep, out of ignorance and a whole host of unrecognized preconceived notions about psychiatry, psychiatrists, and other parents. That psychiatrists medicated kids for expediency and with a callous disregard for their unique personalities and individual life circumstances. ...
>
> Writing this book changed all that.
>
> Listening to those parents, letting their voices ring out louder than the cultural noise surrounding them, a couple of simple truths have become clear.
>
> They are: That the suffering of children with mental health issues ... is very real. That almost no parent takes the issue of psychiatric diagnosis lightly or rushes to "drug" his or her child, and that responsible child psychiatrists don't, either. And those many children's lives are essentially saved by medication. [10]

Warner discovered that hundreds of thousands of parents didn't medicate their kids to get them into Harvard or to turn them into perfect kids. Instead they did so because they were exhausted, scared, and desperate for something to help their children.

When these children did not function, bad things happened. They kicked out windows, beat their younger sisters with bats and chairs, screamed hateful words at everyone, and refused to go to school.

These parents told Warner that critics think they understand ADHD because their kids are sometimes bored or restless. But these parents emphasized to Warner that the reality of ADHD was so far from such common malaises as to be in another universe. It was like the depression of William Styron and Dick Cavett compared to a transient downturn of a normal adult.

French philosophers such as Jacques Derrida, Michael Foucault, and Roland Barthes, and English critic R. D. Laing argue that madness is socially constructed. Scientologists tout these themes through Hollywood stars such as Tom Cruise and Juliette Lewis. Depression, ADHD, and anxiety are not real, these celebrities argue, but the symptoms of individuals controlled by Big Brother aligned with Big Pharma.

But just as clinical depression is real, so ADHD seems very real in many children, and so is the spectrum of Asperger's syndrome and bipolar disorders. The upshot is that for these therapeutic interventions in children and young adults, we are not witnessing a mass, unjustified experiment on vulnerable beings but a revolutionary breakthrough that allows millions of people to function normally in a very competitive society. Without such drugs, affected people fifty years ago were doomed to low-paying jobs, public support, or institutionalization.

One area that does cause concern is the enormous money being made by pharmaceutical companies and their direct funding of psychiatrists who use these drugs. In *White Coat, Black Hat*, bioethicist Carl Elliott emphasizes that in 2003, the top 10 drug companies made as much profit as the other 490 top Fortune 500 companies.[11] Given 5 million children and adolescents on Ritalin and Adderall, and given thousands of psychiatrists and other physicians monitoring them with drug companies rooting them on, the government needs to fund objective studies to make sure that no long-term damage is occurring and that the most cost-effective drugs are being used.

One long-term study in 2011 finally appeared that showed no "serious cardiovascular events" in children taking Ritalin and Adderall over many years, compared to non-using children.[12] At the same time, due to strict enforcement by the Drug Enforcement Administration, which sets quotas for manufacturers of drugs that can be abused in order to thwart abuse, Ritalin and Adderall, and especially their generic versions, were in such short supply that hundreds of patients complained daily to the Food and Drug Administration that they could not find pharmacies to fill their prescriptions.[13]

■■■

Let's now move into the different territory of not just treating problems of cognitive focus in underachieving children but of *improving it* in normal children. Now we are no longer talking about giving methylphenidate or dextroamphetamine to correct dysfunction in children but giving it to children to enhance functioning. Consider something that looks fairly innocuous: giving normal children Ritalin or Adderall to see if it boosts their cognitive performance. The first item to discuss is that this is going to be an experiment. The justification for underperforming kids is the quasi-emergency of lack of progress in school and underdevelopment of the young brain, but in normal kids, this justification vanishes. Second, because children are below the age of consent and vulnerable to the wishes of parents, they need extra protection from overzealous parents. This is precisely the worry that fuels critics of kids presently on methylphenidate and dextroamphetamine.

It is not clear whether the National Institutes of Health or any IRB would allow such experiments. Although research might be allowed on competent adults, it is not clear that it could be done on normal children or adolescents. If so, it is difficult to see how we are going to prove that these drugs improve cognitive performance in children.

Let's return to the issue of enhancements and cheating: is it cheating for subnormal children to become normal with Ritalin? Is it cheating for normal kids to become superior with methylphenidate or dextroamphetamine?

Somehow our intuitions differ here. While it does not seem to be cheating to give subnormal kids Ritalin to allow them to function normally, it does seem like cheating to give normal kids Ritalin to allow them to function supernormally.

Suppose giving normal children Ritalin improves their history test scores by 10 percent. Is this permissible? Answers may depend on how one sees the purpose of education.[14] If it is to allow the talented to win admission to the best schools, prizes, and scholarships, then students using Ritalin to boost scores is cheating. Why? If this drug is not equally available to all test-takers, those scoring the tests will likely assume that all test-takers were free of brain-boosting drugs. Also, we can assume that test-takers will not reveal such usage to those who judge their achievements. In such cases, using Ritalin secretly is cheating.

Moral questions here slide into the larger area of public policy, so we now need to address two related moral issues about giving all children Ritalin: first, will there be an arms race of cognitive enhancers for success in school?

Here is one case where this arms race objection proved false. We do not find an additional million kids on Ritalin with parents hoping that this drug will create superior results in their children. Parents of normal kids appear quite content to refrain from unnecessarily putting their kids on drugs. Let us be thankful for that!

And it's easy to see why. Most parents want the best for their kids, and starting any child on a drug, especially one that modifies his or her brain, is a significant undertaking. Double down on that for putting a child on a drug that may need to be taken for life.

Second, if we wanted to give normal kids Ritalin to raise performance, questions arise of distributive justice: if these tools work, should we give them to the needy first? Should we give Ritalin or modafinil first to high school students who apply to college but score low on standardized tests, see if they improve, and then admit them? Rich kids may get both Kaplan courses and Ritalin, thus exacerbating existing inequalities.

The answer to this objection seems simple: the least-advantaged children are already on methylphenidate and dextroamphetamine. They are the 5 to 7 million. For once, Rawlsian justice is satisfied and we are not seeing cognitive mediations used to exacerbate mental differences in kids of different economic classes.

Alarmists argue that just because we allowed rich parents to buy test-preparation courses for their children, we should now allow them to buy brain-boosting drugs. Can't we draw an ethical bright line somewhere? When it comes to brain enhancements, is the real danger that rich kids will be even more advantaged than now?

These are interesting objections, in part because on most college campuses, Ritalin and Adderall are the most commonly sold or swapped drugs used by normal students before tests or to write long-delayed term papers. As with the use of steroids in male sports and excessive cosmetic surgery in women, a subculture exists where thousands, and maybe millions, of people self-experiment with enhancements and we know little about what's going on. Perhaps it creates more inequality, perhaps not. It's another epistemic black hole. In the final chapter, I will address how to fill this hole.

NOTES

1. British Medical Association, "Boosting Your Brainpower: Ethical Aspects of Cognitive Enhancements," November 2007. (Discussion paper) http://www.bma.org.uk/ethics/health_technology/CognitiveEnhancement2007.jsp#.TyQRpa4-lG4

2. St. Louis Psychologists and Counseling Information and Referral, "ADD: Help is On the Way," http://www.psychtreatment.com/adhd.htm

3. Laurence Diller, *Running on Ritalin: A Physician Reflects on Children, Society and Performance* (New York: Bantam, 1998).

4. Center for Drug Evaluation and Research, Food and Drug Administration, "One Year Post-Pediatric Exclusivity Post-Marketing Adverse Event Review Drug Utililization Analysis," June 20, 2007, pdf document.

5. N. Volkow and J. Swanson, "The Action of Enhancers Can Lead to Addiction," *Nature* 2008 (Jan 31, 2008), 451 (7178): 521.

6. National Alliance Against Mandated Mental Health Screening and Psychiatric Drugging of Children, "Death from Ritalin: The Truth Behind ADHD."http://www.ritalindeath.com/

7. James Hughes, *Citizen Cyborg: Why Democracies Must Respond to the ReDesigned Human of the Future* (Boulder, CO: Westview Press, 2004), 37.

8. Laurence Diller, *Running on Ritalin*.

9. Roni Caryn Rabin, "Drugs to Treat A.D.H.D. Reach the Preschool Set, " *New York Times*, October 25, 2011, D5.

10. Judith Warner, *We've Got Issues: Children and Parents in the Age of Medication* (New York: Riverhead Books, 2010), 2-3.

11. Carl Elliott, *White Coat, Black Hat: Adventures on the Dark Side of Medicine* (Boston: Beacon Press, 2010).

12. William Cooper et al., "ADHD Drugs and Serious Cardiovascular Events in Children and Young Adults," *New England Journal of Medicine*, 365, no. 20, November 17, 2011, 1896–2204.

13. Gardiner Harris, "F.D.A. Finds Short Supply of Attention Deficit Drugs," *New York Times*, December 31, 2011, A1.

14. Anders Sandberg, "The Use of Cognitive Enhancing Drugs: Brain Boosting and Cheating in Exams: Four Responses," *Practical Ethics*, May 22, 2008. http://www.practicalethicsnews.com/practicalethics/2008/05/brain-boosting.html

PART III

CHANGING HUMAN NATURE?

Chapter Fifteen

How *Not* to Think about Genetic Enhancement

In my first chapter, I mentioned that Alarmist biologist Rollin Hotchkiss from Rockefeller University predicted in 1965 that "in five years" parents would be able to order children with blonde hair, blue eyes, and fair skin.[1] Since then, a glittering parade of Alarmists, from Jeremy Rifkin to Leon Kass, wailed that earth-shaking Eugenic choices lurk right before us.

In this chapter, I discuss a new rule for analysis in bioethics, especially analysis of genetic enhancements: respect complexity. The chapter's message is that Enthusiasts for genetic enhancement were premature, but as might be expected, not for the reasons cited by Alarmists.

To begin, consider designer babies. Much discussion of this topic is imaginary and factually inaccurate. Both champions and critics assume that simple changes could be made with relatively few risks and that the main problems are psychological, such as unrealistic expectations of parents or objectifying children as designed commodities.

On the scale of possible harms to babies, those psychological problems are minor. We don't want to try to perfect babies and get dead ones. That's the real ethical problem.

In 2002, Francis Collins, the head of the Human Genome Project, testified before the President's Council on Bioethics, which then held hearings on the ethics of human enhancement.[2] It must have been a fascinating day to discuss that topic because Leon Kass, the arch-critic of enhancement, chaired that Council. The Council contained other members with similar sentiments such as Johns Hopkins political theorist Francis Fukuyama and Harvard political philosopher Michael Sandel. All three either had, or would soon publish, books claiming that human enhancement would tear apart our social fabric or (in Fukuyama's terms) render us "post-human."[3] They argued that we had never done anything like this before, that even the smallest improvement would put us on the slope to Eugenics.

Question: what did Collins tell this Council, and through it, most bioethicists? He first showed the Council a clip from the movie GATTACA, emphasizing what the geneticist said to Antonio and Maria, a couple planning a genetically-selected child (versus their naturally-conceived child, Vincent):

"Your extracted eggs Maria, have been fertilized with Antonio's sperm and we have performed an analysis of the resulting pre-embryos. . . Naturally, no critical pre-dispositions to any of the major inheritable diseases. All that remains is to select the most compatible candidate. . ."
"You've already specified blue eyes, dark hair, and fair skin. I have taken the liberty of eradicating any potentially prejudicial conditions - premature baldness, myopia, alcoholism and addictive susceptibility, propensity for violence and obesity. . . "
"You want to give your child the best possible start. Believe me, we have enough imperfection built-in already. Your child doesn't need any additional burdens. And keep in mind, this child is still you, simply the best of you. You could conceive naturally a thousand times and never get such a result."[4]

In his testimony, Collins says about this scene:

"You can conceive 1,000 times and never get such a result." (quoting from the scene [sic]) An interesting statement, and actually, it raises a potential problem with this whole scenario because that implies the ability, I suppose, if this was going to happen, to have 1,000 or more embryos to choose from, which is a bit of a biological quandary.
And in fact, that is one of the many ways in which this scenario begins to fall apart scientifically because if you were, in fact, to attempt to try to optimize for ten or twenty phenotypes, as the smooth-tongued counselor here was suggesting, and you consider that each of those phenotypes would probably be influenced by five or ten genes, each of which would have perhaps more than two alleles. You quickly get into a combinatorial problem where lacking a million or better embryos, the ability to actually do this in a fashion that gets you very far is pretty limited.

Of course, that's only a small part of the scientific arguments because the concerns of trying to optimize offspring, if they are predicated on this kind of scenario, assume a degree of genetic determinism that we know is not correct, and it will not become correct just because we get smarter about genetics.
Just because we understand the nature part of the nature/nurture equation doesn't mean that the nature part becomes quantitatively more important. It just means we understand it better.

If you understand what Collins told the Council here, you understand the foolishness of all the worries about designer babies and about choosing traits to create perfect babies.

To put this point differently, the complexity of interactions among genes, and between genes and proteins, and among all these and variable environments, is stunningly vast. So to *reliably* produce a beautiful, bright, genetically healthy child with an optimistic personality and musical talent would require life-long experiments in gestating and raising thousands of nearly similar embryos. Such experiments will not occur, in part because they cannot be ethically justified. And without those experiments, we won't know what we're doing in altering genes.

What about trying to change genes after the embryo is formed or in fetal development? This problem of *insertional mutagenesis* plagues most gene therapy. Because we don't understand how to use a virus to insert genes exactly where we want, inserting genes this way often has disastrous consequences.

Even when we could prevent a child from having a devastating condition, say by deleting the genes for Huntington's, we might inadvertently give it cancer. It is not like taking a bad brick at the bottom of a brick wall and replacing it with a good one: it's more like taking it out and leaving a hole, making the whole wall wobble.

Once upon a time, scientists saw genes as preformed traits, with each gene containing built-in instructions for its expression. Now we know the picture is much more complex: that genes interact with each other, that DNA can be unstable, and that how they code for proteins matters greatly in their expression.

A single gene will rarely be responsible for a desirable human trait. Instead, most desirable traits will involve several genes interacting with several environmental factors. The exact features of a particular trait will depend on many environmental inputs that activate specific combinations of genes at key nodes in fetal and child development.

Human fetal development can be seen as traveling down a long road with many forks to get to the final destination, the newborn child. Embryonic development goes down the road a ways to a fork with diverging paths, going one way and not another, and then it moves to dozens of other forks, each with more diverging paths. At each juncture, it travels down only one path to a particular destination (what genetics call the "phenotype" or final characteristics).[5] At each fork, the fetus–baby–developing-child continuum is bombarded with environmental inputs that affect the expression of its gene-package.

To say we know how to order one particular destination and one particular combination of multi-gene, special traits implies that we have already gone down all these forks and paths and studied how millions of embryos each became a specific phenotype. *GATTACA* falsely implied that we can easily know just which embryo to select to get a hirsute male with perfect pitch and optimistic mood.

All of this should make us pause before we insert genes through viruses randomly into human cells, much less crazy talk of trying to make permanent changes in the germ line of future humans.

Were this not complex enough, let's emphasize an important ethical fact about improving humans that makes our subject differ from research in traditional genetics: *we cannot experiment on human fetuses the way animal breeders do with livestock.* We breed generations of dogs for specific traits by controlling which male and female dogs breed with each other and culling unwanted pups from the line, but we cannot do so with humans.

Most human traits will begin with a biological basis in several genes and develop after complex interactions with environmental factors during gestation, infancy, and childhood. For these reasons, predicting what traits a child might exhibit, at a counseling session or from a genetic catalog, will be next-to-impossible.

Some might think the above discussion unduly pessimistic, but consider what happened in gene therapy over the last fifteen years. In 1999, in Tucson, Arizona, seventeen-year-old Jesse Gelsinger heard about experimental gene therapy at the University of Pennsylvania for his inherited disorder, ornithine transcarbamylase deficiency (OTC).

In the genetic disease OTC, the liver doesn't properly cleanse blood of ammonia produced in normal metabolism, resulting in toxic levels. Many OTC newborns die around birth; half don't live to age five. A new regimen of drugs and diet had enabled Jesse to live to be a teenager, but without a cure, OTC would eventually kill him.

Jesse entered the study as a healthy research volunteer. According to a friend, he "wanted to prove he was a man."[6] Penn researchers claim Jesse was informed that the experiment wouldn't help him and told him that it might help OTC babies. His father said Jesse wanted "to help save lives."

So Penn researcher James Wilson sought adults with OTC whose livers still functioned. He injected them with an adenovirus that contained copies of the gene lacking in OTC patients.

Rick Weiss, the former science reporter for the *Washington Post*, reports the grim reality of what actually happened:

> Four days after scientists infused trillions of genetically engineered viruses into Jesse Gelsinger's liver ... the eighteen-year old lay dying in a hospital bed at the University of Pennsylvania. His liver had failed, and the teenager's blood was thickening like jelly and clogging key vessels while his kidneys, brain, and other organs shut down.[7]

The wrongful death lawsuit claimed that Wilson knew the virus had injured other OTC adults and that Wilson failed to use simple, direct language to explain his dangerous study. As University of Pennsylvania bioethicist Arthur Caplan said,

> Not only is it sad that Jesse Gelsinger died, there was never a chance that anybody would benefit from these treatments. They are safety studies. They are not therapeutic in goal. If I gave it to you, we would try to see if you died, too, and if you did, OK.
>
> If you cured anybody, you'd publish it in a religious journal. It would be a miracle. All you're doing is you're saying, I've got this vector. I want to see if it can deliver the gene where I want it to go without killing or hurting or having any side effects.[8]

Wilson only reported to the FDA 39 of 700 problems about the virus, although laws required reporting all. Researchers concluded in 2000 that adenoviruses should only be used as a last resort. After a congressional hearing on Jesse's death, the National Institutes of Health (NIH) vowed to better monitor medical research. It soon stopped Wilson's research at Penn and halted most research on gene therapy.

Between 1999 and 2002, an experimental gene therapy for x-Severe Combined Immunodeficiency Syndrome (x-SCID), the "bubble boy disease," on seventeen French children restored their immune systems. Later, three of the cured children got leukemia and one died, hardly a great success, so officials halted this trial.[9]

In 2007, Jolee Mohr, a thirty-six-year-old woman in Arkansas with mild arthritis enrolled in a gene therapy experiment and died immediately. The inserted genes in the virus allowed a common fungus to grow in her abdomen, which when it became the size of a football, killed her.

In sum, fifteen years of hundreds of experiments in gene therapy have yielded little success.

■■■

So far I have stressed the failures of changing genes to cure current genetic diseases, the complexity of the tasks ahead, and as a result of these two, the huge complexity and risks of attempting to *genetically* enhance humans, either on a one-person basis or for all descendants.

Let's return to the day when Francis Collins told Kass' Bioethics Council that the "ethics community" was wasting its "energies" worrying about genetically enhancing humans. Of enormous importance, Collins testified that with neither germ-line nor somatic therapy scientists lacked the knowledge to conduct safe, human trials on genetic enhancement. Had he wanted to, Francis Collins could have also mentioned the dismal failures of human gene therapy over the previous fifteen years, but was too politically savvy to do this.

Collins delivered his coup de grace when he testified that every conceivable good use of gene enhancement for babies could be done simply, in those couples at high risk, by having them use in vitro fertilization, testing of various embryos for genetic disease (PGD), followed by implantation of healthy embryos without that disease. Nothing else, he said, would be medically needed for decades.

One then wishes one could have been a bioethicist-fly-on-the-wall when he specifically critiqued Alarmist bioethicists, saying they should expend "their energies" elsewhere. But in this case, Collins wasn't preaching to the choir, but testifying before critics who had long since made up their minds. From their subsequent writings, none of them understood what he said.

Even if we overcame these problems and did such large-scale experiments on human children, it would be decades before we knew the results. Clearly, this is never going to happen because America will not experiment on embryos and children this way, because thousands of women will not volunteer to gestate such babies, and because thousands of parents will not agree to raise such babies in similar ways.

As Collins explained these things, it would have been interesting to know what Kass, Fukuyama, and Sandel felt. Did they think that their books had been unethically Alarmist? Did they worry about making the public worry about problems that would not emerge for centuries? Did they worry that their Alarmism might divert the public from solving ongoing, present problems? Probably not.

What we do know is that the *Report* issued the next year by Kass's Council lumped together all kinds of ethical issues about human enhancement and got it terribly wrong.[10] Both the Council and its *Report* could have done so much better, but not only did it do nothing to help, it created unnecessary problems by tilting at windmills.

The lesson here resembles the one from the history of bioethics: separate cases by type and don't lump everything together. By all means, keep simple cases simple, such as letting competent adults try relatively safe practices. On the other hand, appreciate complexity and do not discuss the irreducibly complex as if it were simple. The new rule: keep complex cases complex; don't make them simple.

For all these reasons, genetic enhancement of fetuses, of newborns, of existing individuals, much less future humans, is not going to be feasible, either practically or ethically, for many decades. In this case, both Enthusiasts and the Alarmists were wrong: Alarmists to warn against things that will not be, Enthusiasts to too-eagerly embrace genetic change.

NOTES

1. Rollin Hotchkiss, quoted by Ronald Kotulak, "And Now Your Child Built to Order: Day of Genetic Engineering Near, Biologist Says," *Chicago Tribune*, August 18, 1965, 5.
2. Francis S. Collins, "Genetic Enhancements: Current and Future Prospects," December 13, 2002, Transcript, President's Council on Bioethics.
3. President's Council on Bioethics (Leon Kass, Chair), Leon Kass, *Beyond Therapy: Biotechnology and the Pursuit of Happiness- A Report of the President's Council on Bioethics*, (New York, Dana Press, 2003); Francis Fukuyama, *Our Posthuman Future: Consequences of the Biotechnology Revolution* (New York: Farrar, Straus & Giroux, 2002); Michael Sandel, *The Case Against Perfection: Ethics in the Age of Genetic Engineering* (Cambridge, MA: Harvard University Press, 2007).
4. GATTACA script, Internet Movie Script Database (IMSDb), http://www.imsdb.com/scripts/Gattaca.html

5. Lenny Moss, *What Genes Can't Do* (Boston: MIT Press, 2002), 188.

6. Richard Jerome, "Death by Research," *People Magazine*, February 21, 2000, 123.

7. Deborah Nelson and Rick Weiss, "Hasty Decisions in the Race to a Cure? Gene Therapy Proceeded Despite Safety, Ethics Concerns," *Washington Post*, November 21, 1999, A1.

8. Center for Genetics and Society, "Gelsinger Wrongful Death Lawsuit names Bioethicist Caplan," *Genetics Crossroads Newsletter*, October 16, 2009. http://www.geneticsandsociety.org/article.php?id=2857

9. http://www.scienceonline.org/cgi/content/full/307/5715/1544a

10. President's Council on Bioethics, *Beyond Therapy*.

Chapter Sixteen

Five Psychosocial Objections to Enhancing Genes

In the considerable literature about the ethics of human enhancement, like the considerable literature about human cloning, very few objections concern physical safety to the child. Instead, most raise psychosocial and political objections. This chapter discusses this kind of objection.

As such, one might wonder why I discuss it at all. In putting all forms of human enhancement in the same rigid box, critics make the classic mistake in bioethics. Nevertheless, reviewing these criticisms will allow me to make some useful points, as well as reminding us why different kinds of enhancement should be discussed separately. In the following, I discuss five objections to human enhancement: the Gifts Objection, Changing Human Nature, the Nazi Researcher objection, the Designer Children objection, and the Unjust Objection.

The Gifts Objection: Michael Sandel, a self-labeled liberal political scientist and member of Kass' Bioethics Council, believes that many of the typical arguments against enhancement don't work. Specifically, he thinks that arguments about inequality and safety will not stand. On the other hand, in *The Case Against Perfection* (2007), he argues that one argument does: that we should not attempt to enhance humans because in doing so, we will lose the "giftedness" of human life.

Sandel argues that special gifts in children bring "three key features of our moral landscape—humility, responsibility, and solidarity."[1] Without the sense that life has these gifts, we would be impoverished, left with "nothing to affirm or behold outside our own will."[2] Sandel claims his notion of talents-as-gifts is not religious, much less indebted to religious views that accept the corrupted nature of humans. Nevertheless, he certainly builds on these views.

Even so, I don't think the three values follow in the way he thinks they do. In order to feel solidarity with fellow humans, why do some need to suffer and others have natural gifts? Why can't we feel solidarity while enjoying equal happiness? Why can't the value of responsibility be expressed in choosing against genetic disease? Famous psychologist Nancy Wexler, whose mother died of Huntington's disease and who helped to discover the gene for it, declined to have children (when we lacked a test for Huntington's) in fear that her child might have it. Why wasn't Nancy just as responsible as another woman who raised a child with special needs?

As for humility, it is the paradigmatic Christian virtue, the one that ancient Greeks considered a vice, and the opposite of the master Christian vice, pride. Yes, genetic disease and lack of gifts make people humble, but is being humble a virtue in any world other than a religious one? Why should everyone be humble? Has humility ever helped a great surgeon take risks? Do humble scientists improve humanity?

What about the nonreligious argument? Do we need cavities and rotting teeth to appreciate good teeth as gifts? If fluoridated water has made good teeth seem normal, isn't it better for every child to have good teeth than for a few to have a gift? Do we need disease to appreciate health? Dullards to appreciate wit?

University of Pennsylvania professor Anita Allen decided to raise a child with catastrophic mental illness, and reviewing Sandel's book helped her pinpoint how being against genetic improvement of humans expressed supportive values for parents like her.[3] Modern disability advocates fear that increased choice over the traits of children will lead to less tolerance, less funding, and less appreciation for parents like Professor Allen.

But should this fear-based view guide public policy? Does the desire to improve humans heap scorn on the unfortunate? Does a desire to cure disease mean contempt for the sick? I don't think so. If anything, familiarity with these conditions drives some to try to cure them. When Doug Melton, a Howard Hughes Fellow at Harvard, discovered that his own children had juvenile diabetes, he switched his research toward curing diabetes with embryonic stem cells.[4] Similarly, a scientist whose child died of Batten's disease devoted his career to curing this disease.[5]

Changing Human Nature. A second kind of psychosocial objection to all attempts at human enhancement is that we will pervert our essential natures. Francis Fukuyama wrote in *Our Postmodern Future* that by toying with various enhancements, such as giving growth hormones to short children, we push toward the point of no return. In reading his book, we eagerly awaited his discussion of this key human essence, and we were disappointed when he revealed that this essence was the mysterious "X Factor." Rather than admit that no human essence exists, Fukuyama steadfastly claims that it cannot be described. The classically trained Fukuyama borrowed here from Aristotle, who faced a similar problem in describing the telos of the universe. Wanting to avoid anthropomorphism, Aristotle called it "X."

So Fukuyama gives us the X Factor, but it is a factor that cannot bear the heavy load assigned to it. Because if this essence is so dear to our identity, to our humanity, to our ideals, and our very nature, shouldn't 2,000 years of thinking about it have gotten us a little clearer about what it is?

Fukuyama also argues that if we allow some humans to enhance themselves, we risk upheavals in societies premised on equal human rights. In making some humans greater than others, we undermine human political equality.

Fukuyama here mistakenly assumes that moral human equality depends on claims of factual human equality. Fukuyama fears the instant *Ubermensch* trampling democracies, like Napoleon returning as Arnold Schwarzennegger and, like the latter, getting himself elected.

But equal human rights do *not* depend on humans being equal in something such as intelligence, strength, or wisdom. Humans vary greatly, but their moral worth does not. Indeed, if it did, wouldn't people with *greater* amounts of Factor X logically deserve *greater* rights?

A final false worry is seen in the views of a reviewer of some books on enhancement who charge transhumanists with failing to "reckon with the fact that the same limits that make life difficult also give it meaning."[6] To use the reviewer's examples, if you could get stronger muscles by taking a drug, have youthful sex through sixty years of a relationship, and make yourself less empathetic in certain situations, this would change what it means to be human.

I think that is a little bit true, but the fallacy comes in the slide from "meaning as a human now" to "meaning as a human later." In one sense, a lot of the meaning in my life as a university professor comes from the existence of books, classes, meetings with faculty, and talking to students face-to-face, as well as working on a campus. Without them (working entirely on-line without books) I could still be a professor, but the meaning of my life would differ. So in one sense, meaning for humans changes all the time as history moves on, and in another sense—so long as we raise children to replace us, eat food, and die—its core meaning does not.

Nazi Researchers. A third objection comes frequently: any time anyone raises the subject of improving humans, critics play "the Nazi card." (In ethics debates, members of the audience sometimes guess how long it will be before someone raises such a Nazi Objection. It is called "Godwin's law."[7])

With enhancement, they accuse researchers of being like Eugenic researcher Josef Mengele. However, Mengele's crimes would be even worse if humans could never improve because of his deeds. So we need to understand the real causes of his research, and separate them from modern research, else this objection will stop all progress in ethics.

Mengele heinously experimented on humans. In trying to create blue eyes, he injected blue dye into children's eyes; to see if twins could be produced, he forced female twins to engage in coitus with male twins. He interchanged blood of identical twins to see what happened.

What is common to Mengele and some modern researchers is ambition. It is false that most medical researchers drive themselves hard for love of humanity. Such researchers compete fiercely for large grants, for esteem among their peers, and for fame in the public eye. Anyone who reads the biography of Christiaan Barnard, who performed the first human heart transplants in 1967, will realize how much ambition drove him. A similar desire can be seen in Leonard Bailey, who performed the first xenograft from a baboon named Goobers to a baby named Fae, or William DeVries, who implanted the ill-fated Jarvik-7 artificial heart into a half-dozen patients. This is what drove James Wilson to kill Jesse Gelsinger in attempting to cure a genetic disease.

So we must be wary of ambition among modern researchers, and if researchers were now racing to create the ideal human, we should be worried. However, we are not in such a race, and indeed, were some physicians to attempt such a race, they would be loudly denounced. That is the current state of things.

What is not similar to Nazi Eugenics is that we do not live in a culture of pervasive racism. I know that some critics disagree, but I believe they are wrong. We need only look at the Armed Forces in the United States to see how blacks, Hispanics, gay men, and lesbians have been successfully integrated. Modern life in developed countries remarkably respects diversity, a progress that is truly astounding and one largely unappreciated by today's youth. One need only read about Henry Ford's denouncement of "Jew bankers" for causing World War I, or Theodore Roosevelt's tirades against "yellow niggers" from the Orient, to realize how far we have come. No one could say such things and run for president today, much less could an African-American man be elected president like Barack Obama.

Designer Children. A fourth popular objection to all attempts to enhance children is that badly motivated parents will desire designer children.

For example, in England, about 7 percent of children attend private schools. The cost of such private schools in 2008 for one child came to about $330,000.[8] That is an extraordinary amount of money, and that so many parents pay it shows the willingness of both parents to sacrifice for their children and of their desire to give their children a leg up in life. That children do get a leg up by attending such schools is shown by the fact that most of England's politicians, writers, journalists, and lawyers attended them.

For the sake of this objection, assume that we obtain reliable knowledge about which package of genes create which desirable traits. Or more realistically, assume we have some knowledge about which bundle of traits can be made more likely to occur and how to avoid children with undesirable, gene-based diseases and conditions. If so, would a superior class of children and humans eventually emerge?

Under such assumptions, critics worry that enhancement of humans will create "Superiors" whose abilities will be so far beyond ordinary humans that they will come to dominate them. Here's a start to refuting this silly fear.

First, people will likely be enhanced by degrees in specific ways, not in all-or-nothing, sudden jumps. When children are enhanced, trade-offs will occur. A family of mathematicians nurturing a young Paul Erdös may emphasize math games and proof pyrotechnics, but also inadvertently select for anti-social sentiments.

Second, adolescents who reach puberty will probably not create children with other enhanced people because they will mate for reasons of sex, love, marriage, and status. Insofar as genes ground desirable qualities over two or three generations, they will be rapidly diluted in procreation among those enhanced. That is, the trait will quickly regress to the mean, as enhanced people's children and grandchildren revert back to normal. Indeed, this regression to the mean and our normal procreative liberty shows the difficulty of making *permanent* enhancements in free societies, as most enhanced people will not mate only with other enhanced people, just as most lawyers don't mate with other lawyers.

Third, for the sake of argument, assume some Superiors did emerge. Why assume they would harm humanity? Suppose that graduates of Princeton outperform ordinary college graduates. Should we infer that Superior Princeton graduates will harm humanity? Why assume that Superiority means domination? Physician Paul Farmer went to Duke and Harvard Medical School and founded Partners in Health to serve medical needs in Haiti, Peru, Rwanda, and Russia. Bill Gates created a product the world needed and used his profits to combat HIV and malaria. Superior people will be diverse, with many different goals. We should not impose comic book stereotypes on them.

Another false worry is that parents will stop being good parents with unbounded love for children, but turn into demanding purchasers of designer children whom they view as commodities. In its crudest form, this is Alarmism 101 about genes, choice, and children.

Why is this view incorrect? Let me count the ways.

First, parents love their children, even when fate brings them children with unexpected problems. Parents feel responsible even when random genetic roulette gives their children disastrous genetic conditions. Some scholars think we are hardwired from evolution to respond this way, which explains why we all go mushy when we see someone's new baby.

Second, parents will most likely not be picking a child as a package but looking for specific traits. If selection of traits becomes possible à la *GATTACA*, the informed consent document will specify that unexpected traits may come with the desired trait, that things may not go as planned, and that how the parents raise their child in a specific environment will affect which genes are expressed.

Furthermore, we need some insight into where the attitude came from that parents should be open to love whatever child fate decrees. In the past, parents had no control over any traits of their children, so this attitude gave value to what had to be. It is like coping with cancer by saying that I must have it for a reason, perhaps to grow as a person.

But just as reliable contraception changed attitudes about pregnancy and parenthood, so reliable choices about traits will change attitudes to accepting fate. Insofar as Alarmism has merit, this is its weightiest charge against parental choice, for surely, isn't having parents accept with unconditional love any child that comes along the best overall policy for children?

This is a complex question, but the answer has to be a bit tough-minded. Consider children who are damaged by the actions of physicians, say anoxia during delivery resulting in cerebral palsy. Should parents just accept the damage to the resulting child or should they seek compensation?

Is it best for the child if they do? Perhaps not. It would likely be in the best interest of the child if the parents did not focus on the injury and accept fate. But for future children, it would be better for them to sue to prevent similar injuries.

Similarly with genetic choice. Remember, we are assuming here that we have some reliable knowledge about which traits of children might be gene-based. Even though children are not commodities, parents will, in fact, become less accepting over decades.

Another false worry is that if we enhance some specific traits, our society will come to scorn people with disabilities. But our society is a mansion with many rooms. As some children reach new heights in playing the cello, others without any musical ability will not necessarily suffer. The educational system needs to help each child flourish in his or her own sphere, not impose a one-size-fits-all template.

Besides, people will be enhanced in many ways and for many different reasons. Some enhancements will fail, some will be partially successful, and some will work but be hidden. So much of past enhancements are associated with Eugenics and its blatant public manipulations that we may have a hard time conceiving how private reproductive decisions will have incremental effects and hardly be noticed. Nor is it likely, like some rough beast crouching towards Jerusalem, that changes will sneak up and suddenly one day overwhelm us. Instead, as with intermarriage, almost all small changes will be wiped out in the gene intermingling of subsequent generations.

Improvements in children will also be incremental, in part because some enhancements will be experimental and require approval of ethics committees, the Food and Drug Administration, and the physicians who help bring them about. Some may need public consensus, such as raising a generation of kids on Ritalin, Adderall, or modafinil. Such improvements will take time to evaluate, maybe decades. Most likely, enhancing children will not be a slippery slope, but a long, slow, uphill grind, like the Romans building a dirt road up to Massada. For Vespasian, it took a year. For pediatric enhancement, it may take a century.

So what about the over-discussed example of parents giving short children growth hormones to make them normal? How this is done is very important, both morally and as to whether parents would actually do it. It requires shots with needles three times a week over several years. From this fact, four points emerge: (1) it will be expensive, maybe $20,000 a year, (2) it will require a lot of trips to the hospital or doctor's office, (3) it will probably give the kid a horror of needles and pediatricians, and (4) it has risks, for one contaminated batch of hormone or one contaminated needle could saddle the kid with hepatitis, a neurological disorder, or a bad infection.

Question: What is shared by all descriptions of parents in the Designer Kids Objection? Answer: They all describe bad parents, ones who are selfishly motivated, who are egotistical, and who cannot separate their own narcissism from the separate good of their child. Critics write of such parents as if they all have borderline personalities. In short, critics emphasize both the sinful, fallen nature of man, but also the sinful, selfish, fallen nature of parents. Because humans and human parents are contaminated this way, the dangerous tools of genetic enhancement and biotechnology should be forbidden to them.

Take an example that turns around our intuitions. Suppose a large class of cancers turns out to be viral, and suppose that a generalized vaccine, Preventia, protects kids from it. We can imagine a debate about whether children should be required to get Preventia, but can we imagine legislators who want to criminalize parents who want to give their children Preventia?

Cancer hits generations of some families, leading researchers to believe that some families have a genetic predisposition to cancer. Those families would be especially interested in Preventia, especially if it targeted cancers prevalent in their ancestors. Anyone who has seen the ravages of pancreatic, esophageal, or ovarian cancer can't help but fear these cancers. It is easy to imagine families jumping at a chance to take Preventia, and most would probably take some risks to do so. So woe be to the legislator who would pass a law forbidding parents from giving their children Preventia to prevent cancer.

Notice how this example differs from the ones used by Alarmists, which always involve ambitious parents pushing their kids too hard: tennis moms or parents hiring unemployed professors to prepare their kids' applications to college. Instead of pushy parents, Preventia changes the focus to parents worried about their kids having cancer and shifts the onus of proof: why wouldn't a parent give his or her child insurance against cancer?

In general, remember that we now give parents a lot of freedom in enhancing their kids according to the parents' religious or philosophical views. They can home-school their children and teach them that the Good News Bible or Torah is inerrant, and they can raise them as vegans or Marxists. Giving parents choices isn't necessarily bad.

The Unjust Objection. Finally, the objection exists, as reviewer James Sabin aptly put it, "that the rich will not simply get more—they will become more as well."[9]

Case Western Reserve law professor Maxwell Mehlman argues that no one should be allowed to genetically enhance his brain or body because at first only the rich could do so, and such enhancements will lead to an even more unequal society, a *genobility*.[10] Instead, Mehlman proposes that if anyone at all is enhanced, it should be the genetically least advantaged. Lee Silver in *After Eden* in 1998 suggested that human cloning might one day create a class of GenRich people, far beyond the abilities of present humans.[11]

Mehlman's argument piggybacks on the famous difference principle of John Rawls' theory of justice, in which Rawls argued that structural inequalities in society are only just if they benefit the least well-off groups.[12] Yes, physicians have more powers than ordinary citizens, but this inequality not only benefits average citizens, it should also benefit the neediest citizens. If it does not, if medicine only serves the rich and insured, it is unjust.

A non-Rawlsian, utilitarian argument might also favor enhancing the needy first. Diminishing marginal utility favors enhancing the disadvantaged rather than adding to the powers of the advantaged. If cognitive enhancers could raise the IQ of a child from 70 to 100, we should do that first. A just society would also seem to indicate that, until we elevate all below-normal children, we should withhold enhancers from children with an IQ of 120 and above.

Without the practical details of real contexts, such proposals seem *prima facie* to be fair. Theologian and bioethicist Ronald Cole-Turner wonders whether anyone would object to boosting the intelligence of a person with Down syndrome. [13]

But the reasoning here is like saying that dentists should be banned from putting braces on rich kids with crooked teeth until they fix all broken teeth in poor kids. Writ large, this is the idea of *equalizing up*.

This view has some practical problems. First, consider vulnerable populations in medical research, including the poor, prisoners, and people with disabilities. This has recently been emphasized in research ethics. How would it be justified to start human enhancements, which at first would have to be classified as experimental, on vulnerable people with Down syndrome? Wouldn't it be better to let the most savvy humans assess the possible risks and benefits, then let them volunteer to try the enhancers, rather than using people with Down syndrome?

For example, and to generalize from the results with mice and caffeine, giving adults with Down syndrome five cups of coffee a day might improve their cognitive performance. But the caffeine might also make such people more difficult to handle and interfere with their caregivers' sleep.

Second, even if giving cognitive enhancers to people with Down syndrome were completely safe, how do we overcome the objection that there is nothing wrong with Down people *as they are*? That having the mental ability of a person with Down syndrome is not a deficiency that needs to be enhanced? That if we "fixed" people with Down syndrome, the world would lose people with special viewpoints, gifts, and perspectives?

Third, critics may be misguided in thinking that an enhancement available to most members of society, and which could make them even more advantaged, could be easily transferred to the least advantaged. After their introduction, personal computers eventually became tools that could help the least advantaged, but even now, that is not necessarily so. Some people today still cannot manage the basics of operating a personal computer or a smart phone, much less learning to use a new kind of software.

In *Anarchy, State, and Utopia*, the late Libertarian philosopher Robert Nozick posited a thought experiment to explain how, in the design of a society, liberty can trade off with equality. [14] Suppose, he ventured, that by magic or revolution, every citizen became equal in material goods. What then? How does society keep things equal? People would begin to trade, buy, and sell their goods, and some people would make better trades than others. Over time, the initial equality would be lost.

Were government to forbid trades, equality would remain, but as Nozick argued, forbidding that would require a dictatorship and an intolerable intrusion into personal lives. This is what life has been like in Castro's Cuba.

A similarly horrible situation would develop if, in the name of equality, the state forbade individual self-enhancement of mind, body, or mood. Yes, it sounds fair that we should improve the thought, strength, and mood of the least advantaged people, but even if we overcame the ethical problems of experimenting on them first, there is still the huge problem of how we practically prevent self-enhancement in everyone else. Most suspiciously, we have to prevent parents from trying to give their children genetic advantages. It seems like we would need to have teachers at schools spot any illegally enhanced child and report that child to authorities!

The most intrusive ban, the most egregious threat to personal liberty and autonomy would be a ban on enhancing mood. Although it is a competition of sorts as to whether banning improvements of mind, body, or mood is worst, one's personality and inner feelings of satisfaction are so personal that it's a *reductio ad absurdum* that the state could regulate such private matters. Is the government really going to get into the business of comparing our internal moods and trying to equalize them? Is that its correct role? Should it really prevent a rich person, or one with group medical coverage that will pay for it, from taking modafinil or Prozac?

One of the nice features of separating kinds of cases, and specific subtypes of cases in each major class, is that some things become so clear. We do not really want government to regulate the private moods of competent adults or the desires of parents to advance their children.

Many arguments for a difference principle for genetic justice stem from the category mistake that genetic equality can be measured in dollops and transferred between people to create equal results. This misconceptualizes how genes develop traits and confuses them with transferable things, such as bicycles and barrels of oil. This Transfer Fallacy often occurs in discussions of food policy and relief of famine.[15]

Finally, if it were only a question of which group of people to benefit first, of course we would equalize up and enhance all who suffer from genetic conditions that prevent their equal functioning as humans. But at present, we don't even know which conditions are primarily due to genes, which partly. As I've emphasized, few genetic diseases will turn out to be simplistic scenarios in which those with a certain gene will get a particular disease.

In sum, although the rich can purchase every enhancement and not sacrifice other goods, the marketplace rightly allows middle class and working class individuals to choose to sacrifice for an enhancement for their kids.

Finally, although I think Mehlman's prediction of a genobility is farfetched, and although I think his proposal to impose a genetic difference principle on human enhancement is impractical, I agree that genetic enhancements, if safe and practical, should also be offered to the least advantaged. That does not mean that they should be the first group tested, because they may be the most vulnerable. Especially if public monies finance its development, a just society should also provide an enhancement to the neediest.

In this chapter, I examined five common objections to all human enhancements, and I found them largely baseless. If we don't commit the category mistake in bioethics of classifying everything together, most of these objections sink themselves. Others, as soon as they are closely examined, are so impractical that serious discussion of them makes them collapse. Now that I've dismissed these five common objections, I will move on to the two final chapters that discuss more positive topics.

NOTES

1. Michael Sandel, *The Case Against Perfection: Ethics in the Age of Genetic Engineering* Cambridge MA: The Belknap Press of Harvard University Press, 2007, 86.
2. Michael Sandel, *The Case Against Perfection,* 100.
3. Anita Allen, "Genetic and Moral Enhancement," *The Chronicle Review: The Chronicle of Higher Education*, May 16, 2008, B13ff.
4. "60 Minutes," CBS, June 8, 2008.

5. "A Stem Cell First at OHSU," *The Portland Tribune*, Nov 24, 2006. Batten's disease was the first condition approved by the FDA for injection of purified stem cells into a child's brain in an attempt to restore the ability to walk and talk.

6. Annie Murphy Paul, "'Radical Evolution' and 'More than Human': The Incredibles." *New York Times*, July 3, 2005.

7. http://en.wikipedia.org/wiki/Godwin's_law

8. "Designer Kids," March 2008, *The Economist*.

9. James Sabin, review of Erik Parens, Enhancing Human Traits, *Journal of Health Politics, Policy, and Law*, 26, no. 4, August 2001, 810.

10. Maxwell Mehlman, *Wondergenes: Genetic Enhancement and the Future of Society* (Bloomington, Indiana, Indiana University Press, 2003).

11. Lee Silver, *After Eden* (New York: Harper, 1998).

12. John Rawls, *A Theory of Justice* (Cambridge, MA: Harvard University Belknap Press, 1970).

13. Ronald Cole-Turner, quoted in Bryan Spice, "Creating a 'Genobility,'" *Post-Gazette*, July 16, 2000.

14. Robert Nozick, *Anarchy, State, and Utopia*, New York: Basic Books.

15. Gregory Pence, *Designer Food: Mutant Harvest or Breadbasket of the World?* (Lanham, MD: Rowman & Littlefield, 2002), 152.

Chapter Seventeen

Cloning, Primordial Cells, Enhancement

The last decade has witnessed the birth of potentially spectacular tools for human enhancement. Yet to date, they have not been used maximally. The explanation of this requires some background information.

Stem cells are found in embryos, bone marrow, and the umbilical cord. They help the injured body grow new cells. If the body loses blood, it activates stem cells to make new blood. As primordial cells, stem cells can develop into any kind of differentiated cellular tissue: bone, muscle, nerve, and so forth. In theory, they could be directed to form new bones, neural cells, cardiac tissue, and to cure diseases.

For some time, physicians knew that the human body had stem cells, but they had no easy way to grow them, and tediously derived them from minute amounts of tissue from embryos or fetuses. They were called *embryonic stem cells*.

Then in 1998, John Gearhart of Johns Hopkins University and James Thomson of the University of Wisconsin discovered how to continually produce stem cells—create an immortalized stem cell line. In effect, they discovered how to make human embryos into tiny *stem cell factories*.

Such commodification of cells bothered critics, who felt that using human embryos for such purposes demeaned the dignity of humans and led down a slippery slope.

Gearhart and Thompson made their discoveries using private funds. As such, the ban at the time on the National Institutes of Health's (NIH) funding of research involving human embryos meant that NIH could not fund clinical trials with such embryonic stem cells.

At the time, bioconservatives opposed any research with such cells and indirectly helped discover a different kind of stem cell. In 2001, scientists discovered stem cells not only in bone marrow, but also throughout the human body. Called *adult stem cells,* researchers started using these cells in research rather than using embryonic stem cells. Politically, pundits started to claim that adult stem cells could function just as well as embryonic stem cells.

In the next five years, researchers discovered that many organs and tissues contain precursor cells that act like stem cells. These adult stem cells become specific kinds of cells more quickly than embryonic stem cells.

A director of an institute for regenerative medicine says, "Brain stem cells can make almost all cell types in the brain, and that may be all we need if we want to treat Parkinson's disease or ALS. Embryonic stem cells might not be necessary in those cases."[1] Similar, specific adult stem cells can be obtained from the intestine, skin, liver, and bone marrow.

With heart disease, the director of Harvard's Stem Cell Institute says, "If you could find a progenitor cell in the adult heart that has the ability to replicate, it's likely easier to start with that than begin with an embryonic stem cell, which has too many options."[2]

But most adult organs contain few stem cells, not nearly enough to use medically, and adult stem cells are even harder to grow than embryonic stem cells. More fundamentally, "Unlocking the secrets of self-renewal will most likely involve studying embryonic stem cells," said Harvard's director.

During the presidency of George W. Bush and under Leon Kass' Bioethics Council, Congress tried to make it a federal crime to create or use human embryos for medical research. That meant that such embryos could not be turned into embryonic stem cell factories. Sam Brownback (R–KS) led the fight in the Senate for such a bill, but it did not pass.

Backed by the administration of George W. Bush, a similar proposal to ban all forms of cloning worldwide went before the United Nations but failed. Asian countries such as Korea, Malaysia, and China, hoping to excel in biotechnology, aligned with European countries to resist the measure. Malaysia invested $26 million in its BioValley to house one hundred new biotech companies to work on stem cells and raise Malaysia to a world power in biotechnology.[3] China invested in cloning technology, hoping to gain where the West had stumbled.[4]

With Congress stalemated, action about funding research with human embryos fell to states. In passing Proposition 71, California allocated $3 billion for stem cell research from human embryos. State legislatures across the land then battled to fund or to criminalize embryonic cloning. Wisconsin, New Jersey, Connecticut, Illinois, Washington, Ohio, and Maryland funded research while Arizona, Arkansas, Indiana, Michigan, Oklahoma, and North and South Dakota voted to ban research using cloned human embryos.[5]

In 2009, President Barack Obama gave federal regulators new rules for research with embryonic stem cells. The president created a review panel composed of scientists and ethicists to make sure that the couple whose cells were used to create the embryonic stem cells consented to how their embryos were used. Scientists and the American Medical Association liked the results.

Meanwhile, something more momentous had occurred. Again, opposition to use of embryonic stem cells by bioconservatives indirectly motivated it. In 2007, researcher Shinya Yamanaka of Kyoto University discovered how to use four genes to tell skin cells how to revert back to pluripotent cells, called human iPS cells. Thus he learned how to use a few genes to tell a differentiated somatic cell how to revert back to a primordial state and to become an undifferentiated cell that could turn into anything. Now called induced pluripotent stem cells (iPSCs) or more simply, induced stem cells, these powerful cells appear to eliminate the need for human embryos to create embryonic stem cells.

This was a Nobel-Prize–worthy achievement. Yamanaka proved that induced stem cells can be grown without creating human embryos. He thus bypassed the need for research embryos or eggs from female donors.

In 2009, further progress occurred with induced stem cells. Two Chinese teams created identical mice using embryonic stem cells created from induced stem cells created from the skin of the ancestral mice. This achievement was considered the definitive test in proving that iPS cells can truly function as the equivalent of human embryonic cells.

In 2011, researchers reported in *Nature Cell Biology* that they turned mouse skin cells directly into beating heart cells without the intervening step of creating iPS cells. This is a further stunning advance that leads us to using a person's own cells to grow as medicine for his ills.

Although this achievement appeared to end, or at least, greatly diminish, the controversy over creating human research embryos, it started others. Such cells might be especially valuable in the new field of regenerative medicine.

Using a person's own IPS cells might be the greatest therapeutic innovation in the history of medicine. It may be used to treat bodily dysfunctions and perhaps even to improve functions, jumpstarting the new field of regenerative medicine.

The leading edge of such research is in horses and dogs with bone chips, degenerative arthritis, hip dysplasia, and/or spinal cord injuries. Without the ethical hurdles facing human experimentation, regenerative medicine has made real progress in treating old horses and dogs with these diseases.[6] A San Diego company, VetStem, makes cells out of fat collected from these animals and returns concentrations for injection back into the animals. So far, 80 percent of animals are improved, with only 1 percent having bad reactions.

One day soon, the same will be done for humans, especially those with injuries to the spinal cord or degenerative arthritis. Indeed, the success of the therapy in horses and dogs increases the evidence that such a treatment might work in humans. A mammal is a mammal is a mammal.

According to a recent report on *60 Minutes*, Dr. Anthony Atala of Wake Forest's Institute for Regenerative Medicine has successfully taken bladder cells from several patients' bodies, cultivated them in petri dishes, and layered the results in three-dimensional molds that resemble bladders.[7] Within weeks, the molds began functioning as regular bladders, which Atala then implanted back into patients' bodies. For patients whose ears were severed in accidents, Atala has grown new ears in six to eight weeks and, because the new ears were grown from the patient's own cells, they were accepted by their bodies. Atala has also grown a human heart valve that beats, originated from human cardiac cells. It will start clinical trials in a few years.

Another leading edge of regenerative medicine is at the University of Pittsburgh, where surgeon Dr. Stephen Badylak directs the McGowan Institute for Regenerative Medicine. Badylak seeks to find the body's internal signal to turn pluripotent cells into particular types. Using human embryonic stem cells or their equivalents, Badylak wants to replace parts of human bodies the way newts and salamanders do. He's developed an Extra Cellular Matrix (ECM) that is the platform for replacing various human parts.

We do not yet know how induced stem cells will advance these projects, but they cannot be anything but helpful. For one thing, we don't need eggs of females to create human embryos or, for that matter, human embryos at all.

Badylak's most successful project was growing a new esophagus for a patient with esophageal cancer. When surgeons removed the damaged esophagus, they replaced it with an ECM sleeve of the patient's healthy esophageal cells. Six months later, the patient was cancer-free.

In 2008 at the University of Barcelona, Paolo Macchiarini performed the first tissue engineered trachea transplantation. He took adult stem cells from a patient's bone marrow, grew them into a large population, matured them into cartilage cells, and seeded these with epithileal cells into a purified tracheal segment from a cadaveric donor.

In a promising development, the Australian firm Mesoblast reported "outstanding evidence" that injecting stem cells into the heart of patients with moderate cardiac damage could reduce the risk of further heart attacks by 80 percent.[8] It had similar trials with stem cells in patients with leukemia.

In the military, $250 million goes to fund replacements for burned skin or lost limbs. At the Army's Institute for Surgical Research, surgeons placed ECMs grown from the tissue of injured vets in traumatic leg wounds and successfully prevented amputation. The ECMs took tissue from the vet's remaining leg and grew muscle, allowing the veteran to later walk unaided.

At Pittsburgh, similar ECMs allow veterans who have lost hands to have better hand transplants from cadavers. Surgeons transplanted bone marrow from such cadavers to the veterans, and grafted cells from both patient and donor into ECM, successfully performing a hand transplant without the need of life-long use of toxic, immune-suppressing drugs.

Suppose scientists learn how to quickly grow iPSC cells from an athlete and inject them back into his muscles, immune system, bones, and organs. Suppose these injections increased performance and appeared safe. What should we make of this?

First, note that it voids the unnatural objection. What could be more natural than injecting bits of me back into me? Second, it raises the objection that, as an enhancement in sports, it might be impossible to detect. Because they are my cells with my genes and proteins, they will not be rejected by my immune system and will work with my existing organs. By the same facts, no test is going to mark them as different. Unless a test could be developed for higher concentrations of one's own stem cells or new stem cells in odd places, it would be impossible to prevent such usage in sports.

However, we should not side too much here with Enthusiasm. Caution based on evidence is necessary. James Wilson, whose own research killed Jesse Gelsinger, warns that we should not repeat the errors of gene therapy with stem cells. We should not naively believe we can insert primordial cells into people and that they will instantly morph into helpful cardiac cells. Even if I am injecting my own cells back into me, this could be dangerous. The injection could disrupt my immune system, cause cancer, or even, like the Gelsinger case, kill me. Nothing is ever simple or without risk.

Good science, good facts, and solid evidence must be behind any protocol. However much we want stem cells to be therapeutic, we must first prove them safe in Phase I trials, then test their ability to be therapeutic, and finally test them against existing therapies.

■■■

In conclusion, these are exciting developments: ones at the cusp of a new era not only of regenerative medicine, but also of enhancement. The same techniques used to grow my induced stem cells into cardiac cells to repair a damaged heart might be used before my heart is injured to enhance it.

We now need to embrace this new frontier, fund it, and move ahead. This book concludes with some practical proposals for doing so.

NOTES

1. Arnold Kriegstein, Director, University of California Institute of Regenerative Medicine, quoted in "What A Bush Veto Would Mean for Stem Cells," Nancy Gibbs and Alice Park, *TIME*, July 24, 2006, 36.

2. Douglas Melton, quoted in "What A Bush Veto Would Mean for Stem Cells," Nancy Gibbs and Alice Park, *TIME*, July 24, 2006, 36.

3. Chee Yoke Heong, "Malaysia's New Dream: Biovalley," *Asia Times*, 2003.

4. "China, a Cloning Paradise," *Asia Times*, February 24, 2005.

5. "State Cloning Laws," The National Conference of State Legislators, April 18, 2006. http://ncls.org/programs/health/Genetics/rt-shcl.htm

6. "Stem Cells for Fido," *Nightline*, ABC News, June 24, 2008; "Stem Cell Therapy for Pets," *TIME*, July 7, 2008.

7. "Growing Body Parts," Morley Safer interview, *60 Minutes*, December 14, 2009.

8. Natasha Khan, "Study: Heart Failure May Be Cut with Stem Cells," *Bloomberg News*, December 8, 2011.

Chapter Eighteen

Conclusions and Six Practical Proposals

Despite a barrage of propaganda to the contrary, the last fifty years have not seen great medical progress. Little systematic progress in human enhancement has occurred, and the success that has happened has been sporadic and often financed privately.

With each success, Alarmists moan that we are corrupting our natures, exhibiting narcissism, and falling into Eugenics. Of course, in bioethics it's always safer to criticize than to praise. If you get behind an innovation, it might create unexpected harm, and later, you might be criticized. Better to imply that life is perfect as it is.

Over the last decades, the worst debacle occurred with embryonic stem cells. If the National Institutes of Health had funded translational stem cell research from the start, breakthroughs in medicine would be a decade closer now.

We can't wait on Alarmists to come around to the pro-enhancement position; they never will. (Although when their own children and grandchildren need artificial hips, modafinil, and assisted reproduction, they will certainly use any advances.)

Equally true, we can't be uncritical enthusiasts about new medical technology. Debacles in gene therapy should not be repeated with stem cells. No matter how much we need cures and want to defeat aging, new technologies must be tested in randomized clinical trials where the financial interests of innovators do not bias the results. Too much of experimental enhancement is fueled by desire for profits, without any corresponding oversight.

Overall, progress is a slog. Resistance to vaccinations grows, gene therapy is going nowhere, and steroids, modafinil, and other efforts are tested in secret, with no accountability, transparency, or publicly verified results.

The worst thing we can do, which the media sometimes fosters, is to just sit back and assume that progress will occur: that humans will get better, stronger, live longer and better, and that we need make no changes in how we think about ethics or how we fund human enhancement. This history of progress in medicine, especially where ethical criticism enters, is two steps forward, three steps backward, four steps forward.

With all this in mind, I offer the following six practical proposals to move us forward:

1. CREATE A DATABASE TO STUDY COVERT ATTEMPTS AT SELF-ENHANCEMENT

To have the best base for developing good public policy, we should assemble the most extensive knowledge of past enhancements—chemical, mechanical, pharmaceutical, nutritional, somatic genetic, and germ-line genetic—and understand the forces that brought about good and bad results. We should also understand any unexpected consequences.

Because so much of this has been sub rosa, we need to find a way for citizens to anonymously report what they've been doing. If thousands of athletes secretly take steroids, we need to know about this and find a way to follow them for decades to discover if they've harmed themselves. If thousands of patients regret cosmetic surgery but are too embarrassed to tell anyone, we need to know that. If thousands of college students take Ritalin or Adderall to study for exams, we need to follow that trend.

Consumers Union, Union of Concerned Scientists, where are you? We need an anonymous, confidential way that people and physicians can report both good and bad results.

These efforts must be international. Some enhancement attempts will be conducted offshore and will vary by culture (some cultures will accept enhancement faster than others).

There is a great deal of self-medication going on that we need to know about. Simply walk into any health food store and gaze at the bewildering variety of products sold. St. John's wort is sold as an antidepressant; kava is used to calm the nerves, and there are a range of products for better skin, sexual function, or digestion. As with aspirin (or acetylsalicylic acid, derived from the bark of willow trees), some of these herbs are likely to work. We should have some formal way of knowing how dangerous these herbs are and whether people are wasting their money on them (they are used most by people with little or no medical coverage).

Resistance inside medicine once existed for studying nontraditional medicine. In U.S. medical centers, Western practices were seen as the only good medicine. Gradually, this view weakened. The stunning success of LASIK surgery, long practiced in Russia, showed how blind American ophthalmologists had been.

In the last decades of the twentieth century, physicians learned that patients often took herbs and supplements that might interfere with prescription drugs, and that no one had studied these herbs carefully, nor did a reporting requirement exist about adverse events from using such herbs. As a result, Congress created the National Center for Complementary and Alternative Medicine (NCCAM) in 1998 to study such herbs and supplements. Now, if you want to learn whether the money your aunt spends on chondroitin or glucosamine is wasted, you can click on the NCCAM Web site.[1]

Nevertheless, it is a continuing scandal that Americans may die from a dangerous supplement, and no store or health practitioner is legally bound to report anything about such deaths to any authority. Some European countries do have such requirements, which is why we know that kava caused several patients to lose their livers.[2]

We need a center where people could report adverse events from taking herbs, vitamins, and minerals, as well as from taking steroids, growth hormone, and any other substance not currently covered by laws requiring mandatory reporting. Ideally, this would be an international center. One of its main jobs would be to track the results of millions of people who self-medicate with off-label uses of prescription drugs.

2. CREATE A NATIONAL CENTER FOR HUMAN
IMPROVEMENT

We need a similar site and national center for enhancement medicine, i.e., a center dedicated to improving existing human brains, bodies, moods, and life spans, as well as doing the same for fetuses, newborns, preschool children, and future humans. A National Center for Human Improvement (NCHI) could fund research and pay top scientists to review proposals, like the system used by NIH. Wouldn't it be great to have fMRI studies of caffeine versus modafinil versus amphetamines for effects on mental competition? Memory loss?

Because we always need to follow the money trail in bioethics, we need to ask how pharmaceutical companies could make money in developing cognitive enhancers. One solution is for the U.S. Food and Drug Administration (FDA) and insurance companies to reject the old distinction between therapy and enhancement, and let people get reimbursed for developing enhancing drugs.

Suppose that, for the last century, the U. S. government had been funding not just therapy for damaged brains but brain enhancement. Who knows where we would be now? And who knows how many side benefits might occur from doing so for brain injuries? We could be so much more than we are, if only we had the courage to pursue that vision.

Inside that center, a special place should be reserved for improving humanity through public health. As this book has shown, incremental changes over time in this area will benefit more humans than any sensationalistic changes in our genome.

3. PUBLICLY FUND COMPARISON STUDIES OF DRUGS,
SUPPLEMENTS, AND COSMETIC PROCEDURES

Millions of expectant parents seem to be experimenting on their fetuses with supplements, prescription vitamins, and other activities, such as putting the songs of Baby Mozart on a pregnant woman's tummy. Wouldn't it be nice if someone studied these efforts and reported on them systematically?

In 2012, under a new federal law, Americans will pay $1 to fund "outcomes research" in medicine. Too bad citizens can't fund the same for enhancement medicine. If they had, perhaps French, Brazilian, and Venezuelan citizens wouldn't have to remove 60,000 breast implants filled with substandard, industrial silicone.[3] If they had, after one French woman died from a rare leukemia after her implants leaked, thousands of French women wouldn't be agonizing about whether to remove or replace their implants.[4] French authorities brought criminal charges against the owner of the company making the implants.

Similarly, if physicians must practice outside their training by doing liposuction or facial peeling, let's study whether their results match those of trained surgeons and dermatologists. If they don't, such "practice shift" should be made illegal.

4. IN BIOETHICS, LAW, AND PUBLIC POLICY: USE THE METHOD OF ANALYZING DIFFERENT KINDS OF CASES SEPARATELY AND RESPECT COMPLEXITY

The usefulness of this method is proved by the history of bioethics, by the arguments given, and by the results of this book.

Consider how brilliant Harvard intuitionist philosopher Frances Kamm criticizes Michael Sandel's argument against parents using drugs or genetics to enhance natural gifts of children:

> To the extent which Sandel allows training and appliances to be used to transform gifts, nothing in his argument rules out using drugs or genetic manipulation that do exactly the same thing. So suppose that a certain amount of voice training is permitted to strengthen the vocal chords. Would a drug or genetic manipulation that could strengthen vocal chords to the same degree also be permissible? If the argument Sandel gives does not alone rule out training, it alone will not rule out transformation by drugs or genetic means, because a girl is transformed to the same degree by each method. If appliances such as running shoes are allowed, why not genetically transformed feet that function the same way?[5]

As a logical argument, this reasoning is impeccable *if* the results are exactly the same, *if* the attempts are exactly the same, and *if* the motives are exactly the same, which Kamm seems to assume, but those are huge "ifs." In subsequent sentences, she notes that Sandel may need, and does not give, a special argument that using drugs or genetics to transform capacities has moral significance, i.e., they differ morally in crucial ways from ordinary parental training and influence. But background conditions immediately indicate that these three types of enhancement *do* differ as means of enhancement. Life is messier and more complex than tight, logical categories allow: voice training is slow, requires effort by the child and involvement by parents (taking the child to lessons, finding a good teacher, attending concerts). In contrast, a drug that could strengthen vocal chords "to the same degree" not only lacks these qualities but runs the risk, as all drugs run, of being too-hastily approved by the FDA at the urging of drug companies, of being prescribed too widely off label to the wrong population, and of making children dependent on it. Similarly, a genetic change in the vocal chords, whereas Kamm presumably means a change just in this child's genes and not in her descendants, runs the risk of innumerable things going wrong, none of which justify better vocal chords.

Finally, because children are vulnerable and must suffer the decisions of their parents, the degree of risk inflicted on them *does* matter, especially when medical professionals must administer the risk-taking means. And the different degrees of risk to vulnerable children create a moral difference in the means employed.

I have been teaching about ethical issues for nearly forty years, and I've noticed that beginners often want to discuss a problem too abstractly. It's tempting to think there's one yes-or-no answer to be discovered by thinking about whether enhancing humans is moral or not. But that's almost never a helpful way to approach real-life problems. Real ethical problems usually show us more, rather than less, complexity.

Consider the desire of some parents of Down children to normalize their child's facial appearance through surgery. The eyes and ears of such children can be changed remarkably. Is that an enhancement or does it just normalize children with a defect? One argument for saying the latter is that under that categorization, group medical coverage would be more likely to pay for the operations.

From my viewpoint, such surgery is cosmetic and is enhancing, but if it makes life better for such children and their parents, not only should it be allowed, but group medical coverage should pay for it on Rawlsian grounds.

Recently, CBS News published a story criticizing a program at Duke Medical School that promised cancer patients a personal-genomic chemotherapy.[6] Hailed for five years as a miraculous breakthrough, it turned out to be fraudulent, and how could it not be otherwise? Given our discussion about complexity in chapter 15, and the dangers of hucksterism with personalized genomics in chapter 9, such fraud seems inevitable. To prove that one chemotherapy suppressed tumors better in me than you, scientists would need thousands of tumors, DNA samples, and studies. Those have not occurred, even in animals, and it is a big jump from animals to humans. Given complexity, we will need a country such as Iceland to sell their medical records and DNA of all its citizens, as they did for DeCode Genetics. We will need high-powered computers parsing DNA samples, of the kind used by Craig Venter and Francis Collins in finishing the Human Genome Project. But that is a long time off, and in the meantime, we should learn to beware of simplistic answers to complex questions.

5. SYSTEMATICALLY STUDY ENHANCEMENTS NOW RATHER THAN LATER

I want to make two final pleas here for a *systematic* study of human enhancement: First, there is the argument from a national security viewpoint. Other countries and their intelligence/military branches will undoubtedly employ enhancement techniques to gain an edge. Not all of them are liberal democracies. Can we twiddle our thumbs while others pursue objective knowledge of better bodies, minds, moods, and longevity? Improve the IQ of whole generations of their kids while we debate Alarmists who love us as we are?

Second, contests in the global marketplace will be increasingly won by those who are the smartest, who are the most knowledgeable, and who possess the best tools. During the next century, surely the Pacific Rim will rise to challenge the rest of the world. Already possessing a tremendous work ethic, Asia may surpass everyone.

Already, countries such as Singapore and South Korea pour vast sums into biotechnology. The years under George W. Bush and Leon Kass allowed these Pacific Rim countries to get ahead of us. Will biotechnology be the way North America stays ahead or will its Puritan heritage explain why it failed?

I'm not arguing that we should study enhancement because "it's going to happen anyway." Rather, I'm arguing that others are likely to try to make it happen, and that if we stagnate with Alarmist self-criticism while they do, we won't have the chance to compete and we will be forced to play catch-up in crisis mode. If we embrace it now, we can do it ethically and publicly, not in some covert lab of the armed forces.

6. ELEVATE THE DEBATE BEYOND THE TWO FRAMES STORIES OF ALARMISM AND ENTHUSIASM

Alarmists such as Francis Fukuyama, Leon Kass, Bill McKibben, and Michael Sandel resemble scouts on the U.S. frontier at the time of the Mayflower. They hear rumors of a distant battle with Native Americans, thousands of miles away on a shore across the country; these Alarmist scouts warn us of the dangers of traveling there. Other scouts, Enthusiasts, hear about that shore and eagerly want to go there, pooh-poohing possible dangers along the way.

Meanwhile, as winter approaches back at Plymouth Rock, we're hungry and trying to grow corn, wondering why our scouts aren't helping. We appreciate the good intentions of scouts, for they *think* they're helping us, but wouldn't it be better for all of us if everyone focused on practical steps that we can take right now to help?

Mr. Fukuyama, we don't need to worry about genetics changing human nature because it's not going to be a problem. Genetic experiments on babies will not be allowed because they're dangerous, will be extraordinarily complex to evaluate, and never gain ethical traction. A fortiori, the same goes for experiments that would change the human genome or try to improve it.

Practically, we're going to live longer and better; we already do. Let's embrace it, find ways to distribute it more fairly, study it scientifically, and move forward together.

NOTES

1. http://nccam.nih.gov/ For example, "In a study published in the *New England Journal of Medicine*, the popular dietary supplement combination of glucosamine plus chondroitin sulfate did not provide significant relief from osteoarthritis pain among all

participants. However, a smaller subgroup of study participants with moderate-to-severe pain showed significant relief with the combined supplements." News release, February 22, 2006. http://nccam.nih.gov/research/results/gait/

2. Fu S. et al., "Influence of Kavain on Hepatic Ultrastructure," *World Journal of Gastroenterology* (January 28, 2008), 14, no. 4, 541–46.

3. David Jolly and Maia de la Baume, "France Recommends Removal of Suspect Breast Implants," *New York Times*, December 24, 2011, A6.

4. "Maia de la Baume, "Frenchwomen Worry about Suspect Breast Implants," *New York Times*, January 17, 2101, All.

5. Frances Kamm, "What is and is Not Wrong with Enhancement?" Faculty Research Working Papers Series, John F. Kennedy School of Government, Harvard University, May 2006, RWP06-020, 25.

6. "Deception at Duke: Fraud in Cancer Care?" *60 Minutes*, CBS News, February 12, 2012. http://www.cbsnews.com/8301-18560162-57376073/deception-at-duke/

Bibliography

Altman, Lawrence K. *Who Goes First? The Story of Self-Experimentation in Medicine.* New York: Random House, 1986.

Bailey, Ronald. *Liberation Biology: The Scientific and Moral Case for the Biotech Revolution.* Amherst, NY: Prometheus Books, 2005.

Bova, Ben. *Immortality: How Science is Extending your Life Span and Changing the World.* Avon, 1998.

Callahan, Daniel. *What Kind of Life? The Limits of Medical Progress*, New York: Simon & Shuster, 1990.

Elliot, Carl, and Peter Kramer. *Better than Well: American Medicine Meets the American Dream.* New York: Norton, 2004.

Elliot, Carl. *White Coat, Black Hat: Adventures on the Dark Side of Medicine.* Boston: Beacon Press, 2010.

Evans, John. *Playing God: Human Genetic Engineering and the Rationalization of Public Debate.* Chicago: University of Chicago, 2002.

Fukuyama, Francis. *Our Posthuman Future: Consequences of the Biotechnology Revolution.* New York: Farrar, Straus & Giroux, 2002.

Garreau, Joel. *Radical Evolution: The Promise and Peril of Enhancing Our Minds, Our Bodies, and What It Means to Be Human.* Broadway Books, 2005.

Goodfield, June. *Playing God?* Random House, 1977.

Green, Ronald. *Babies By Design: The Ethics of Genetic Choice.* New Haven, CT: Yale University Press, 2007.

Habermas, Jürgen. *The Future of Human Nature.* London: Polity, 2003.

Harris, John. *Enhancing Evolution: The Ethical Case for Making Better People.* Princeton, NJ: Princeton University Press, 2007.

Harris, John. *Wonderman and Wonderwoman: The Ethics of Human Biotechnology.* New York: Oxford University Press, 1992.

Hughes, James. *Citizen Cyborg.* Boulder, CO: Westview Press, 2004.

Kramer, Peter D. *Listening to Prozac.* Viking Press, 1993.

Leary, Timothy. *The Politics of Ecstasy.* Oakland, CA: Ronin Publishing, 1980.

McKibben, Bill. *Enough! Staying Human in an Engineered Age.* New York: Times Books, 2003.

Moss, Lenny. *What Genes Can't Do.* Bradford Books and MIT Press, 2004.

Olshansky, S. J., and Bruce A. Carnes. *The Quest for Immortality: Science at the Frontiers of Aging*. New York: W. W. Norton, 2001.

Pence, Gregory. *Classic Cases in Medical Ethics: Account of the Cases that Shaped and Defined Medical Ethics*. New York: McGraw-Hill, 2008.

———. *Cloning After Dolly: Who's Still Afraid?* Lanham, MD: Rowman & Littlefield, 2004.

———. *ReCreating Medicine*. Lanham, MD: Rowman & Littlefield, 2000.

———. *The Elements of Bioethics*. New York: McGraw-Hill, 2007.

———.*Who's Afraid of Human Cloning?* Lanham, MD: Rowman & Littlefield, 1998.

Peters, Philip G. *How Safe is Safe Enough? Obligations to the Children of Reproductive Technology*. Oxford, 2004.

Plotz, David. *The Genius Factory*. New York: Random House, 2006.

President's Council on Bioethics. *Beyond Therapy: Biotechnology and the Pursuit of Happiness*. Washington, D.C.: Dana Press, 2003.

Rifkin, Jeremy, and Ted Howard. *Who Should Play God? The Artificial Creation of Life and What It Means for the Future of the Human Race*. 1977.

Sandel Michael. *The Case Against Perfection: Ethics in the Age of Genetic Engineering*. Cambridge, MA: Harvard University Press, 2007.

Shostak, Stanley. *Becoming Immortal: Combining Cloning and Stem-Cell Therapy*. SUNY Press, 2002.

Silver, Lee. *Re-Making Eden: Cloning Beyond in a Brave New World*. Avon Books, 2007.

Stock, Gregory. *Redesigning Humans: Our Inevitable Genetic Future*. Houghton Miflin, 2002.

Stock, Gregory and John Campbell. *Engineering the Human Germline*. Oxford, 2000.

Savulescu, Julian, Ruud ter Meulen, & Guy Kahane, eds. *Enhancing Human Capacities*. London: Wiley-Blackwell, 2011.

Savulescu, Julian and Nick Bostrom, eds. *Human Enhancement*. London: Oxford University Press, 2009.

Walters, LeRoy and Julie Gage Palmer. *The Ethics of Human Gene Therapy*. Oxford, 1997.

Wilson, Eric. *Against Happiness: In Praise of Melancholy*. New York: Farrar, Straus and Giroux, 2009.

Index